Gymnastics

Everything You Need to Know About Gymnastics

(How to train muscles using your body weight)

Arthur Boyer

Published By **Andrew Zen**

Arthur Boyer

All Rights Reserved

Gymnastics: Everything You Need to Know About Gymnastics (How to train muscles using your body weight)

ISBN   978-1-7779885-3-1

No part of this guidebook shall be reproduced in any form without permission in writing from the publisher except in the case of brief quotations embodied in critical articles or reviews.

Legal & Disclaimer

The information contained in this book is not designed to replace or take the place of any form of medicine or professional medical advice. The information in this book has been provided for educational & entertainment purposes only.

The information contained in this book has been compiled from sources deemed reliable, and it is accurate to the best of the Author's knowledge; however, the Author cannot guarantee its accuracy and validity and cannot be held liable for any errors or omissions. Changes are periodically made to this book. You must consult your doctor or get professional medical advice before using any of the suggested remedies, techniques, or information in this book.

Upon using the information contained in this book, you agree to hold harmless the Author from and against any damages, costs, and expenses, including any legal fees potentially resulting from the application of any of the information provided by this guide. This disclaimer applies to any damages or injury caused by the use and application, whether directly or indirectly, of any advice or information presented, whether for breach of contract, tort, negligence, personal injury, criminal intent, or under any other cause of action.

You agree to accept all risks of using the information presented inside this book. You need to consult a professional medical practitioner in order to ensure you are both able and healthy enough to participate in this program.

Table Of Contents

Chapter 1: History Of Gymnastics 1

Chapter 2: Choosing A Gym 3

Chapter 3: 9 Basic Gymnastics Skills You Should Master 8

Chapter 4: Understanding Xcel And Jo Gymnastics Programs 14

Chapter 5: Elite Gymnastics 20

Chapter 6: Gymnastics Scoring Jo, College, Elite And Olympic................................... 29

Chapter 7: The Difference Between Usag And Aau 61

Chapter 8: Other Gymnastics Programs (Tops, Hopes, And Future Stars)............. 64

Chapter 9: Collegiate Gymnastics........... 69

Chapter 10: What Exactly Is A Specialist In Gymnastics?... 106

Chapter 11: Gymnastics Meet Fees...... 120

Chapter 12: The Mental Meltdown...... 131

Chapter 13: Goal Setting Level Of Difficulties... 144

Chapter 14: Thought Suppression Mental Meltdown 156

Chapter 15: Self- Talk........................... 171

Chapter 16: Attention 180

Chapter 1: History Of Gymnastics

The sport of gymnastics was believed to have started in early Greece around 2500 years ago when it was utilized in the training of athletes to ensure they were in shape for sports as well as war. The participants were not there only to play sports but also to learn about music, art as well as philosophy. The Greeks believed that symmetry between body and mind could be achieved only when physical activity was in conjunction with intellectual pursuits. Plato, Homer and Aristotle were ardent supporters of the strength-building benefits of exercise.

Due to their passion for rope climbing, tumbling as well as other sports The Athenians financed the long-running Olympic Games. In the time that the Romans occupied Greece They discovered the importance of gymnastics as a part of their military education. After the demise of the Roman Empire, gymnastics vanished over the course of hundreds of years.

The concept of "artistic gymnastics" emerged in the beginning of 1800s in order to differentiate different styles of free movement from methods used by the military. While it was regarded as a unique practice by many, the sport of gymnastics began taking off at athletic clubs, schools as well as various other organizations throughout Europe during the early 1880s. As the Olympic movement came back to life in Athens in the year 1896, gymnastics became one of the sports that was that was included.

The Olympic programme began to get settled in 1924 with athletes racing for individual medals, and for team events on every apparatus. A few years later, women were able to compete in Olympic gymnastics in Amsterdam.

Chapter 2: Choosing A Gym

Find the nearest gym which has a gymnastics class that will train you up to the level of elite. Prepare yourself to work many hours, and establish realistic targets for you. Be sure to make your time and relax, as well as take care of your body and mind so you don't get burned out!

The top gymnasiums across the nation could not be found within your area. A lot of families relocate across the nation or have gymnasts stay with their host families to attend the best gymnasiums. The best gymnastics programs are run and run by people who have experience competing in Olympic level gymnastics, as well as knowledge of efficient and safe methods of training.

Verify that the facility is affiliated with the country's governing body for gymnastics competitions like USA Gymnastics in the U.S.

The majority of national gymnastics' organisations are associated with FIG

(Federation Internationale of Gymnastics) The international leading body that governs competitive gymnastics.

If you live in the U.S., you can find USA Gymnastics member gyms by using the USA Gymnastics search directory: https://usagym.org/pages/find/gym.html.

The most prestigious gyms are fitted with the latest and secure equipment and facilities, they have a proven track record of putting athletes at the top or Olympic levels, as well as getting athletic scholarships for gymnastics on the college or university levels. As per the "British Journal of Sports Medicine," the best facilities equipped with top-quality equipment, as well as good ability to spot the coach's team are vital to running an effective gym.

Top East Coast Gymnastics Gyms

One of the most renowned gymnastics facilities located in northeastern the New York's Dynamic Gymnastics situated at

Mohegan Lake, New York. It is owned and operated by two ex- Olympians, Sorin Cepoi and Teodora Ungureanu. Dynamic as well as World Cup Gymnastics in Chappaqua, New York, is the sole New York State gym to include members on the U.S. National Team for three years consecutively. Brestyan's American Gymnastics in Burlington, Maine that has was the training ground for Olympic as well as World gold medalist Alicia Sacramone, and Hill's Gymnastics located in Gaithersburg, Maryland, home to three-time Olympian Dominique Dawes, round out the most prestigious East Coast gymnastics facilities.

Top West Coast Gymnastics Gyms

Gymcats located in Henderson, Nevada, and the All Olympia Gymnastics Center located in Los Angeles, California, is sure to be on the list of the best West Coast gymnastics gyms. Gymcats is the place of Olympian Tasha Schwarrt and All Olympia provides training center of 2 U.S. National Team members.

Top Gymnastics Gyms in the Heartland

It is the Great American Gymnastics Express in Blue Springs, Missouri, is among the best gyms of the American heartland. It was also the place for Olympians Terin Humphrey as well as Courtney McCool. The instruction provided by Chow's Gymnastics & Dance Institute led to Olympic winner Shawn Johnson, and in Fairfield, Ohio, Cincinnati Gymnastics was the place to get the coaching which helped Amanda Borden and Jaycie Phelps to achieve success on the both the national as well as Olympic level.

Top Gymnastics Gyms in the South

One of the must-haves on the list of best gymnasiums would be Karolyi Camp located in New Waverly, Texas, managed and owned by Bela and Marta Karolyi. Bela has provided training to numerous top U.S. and international Olympians such as Nadia Comenici, Teodora Ungureanu, Mary Lou Retton, Kerri Strug, Kim Zmeskal and Kristie Phillips. Marta is the U.S. National Team

Coordinator for USA Gymnastics. In Texas is Dreams located in Coppell, Texas, owned by Olympian Kim Zmeskal and National Team participant Chris Burdette, the World Olympic Gymnastics Academy located which is located in Plano, Texas, which has produced Olympians Carly Patterson and Nastia Lukin.

Pro Tip

Make sure you are aware that USA Gymnastics member gyms are bound to follow specific rules to ensure safety and ethical conduct. Request the details of the prospective facility's code of conduct as well as liability insurance details.

Chapter 3: 9 Basic Gymnastics Skills You Should Master

There are specific skills that you can learn in gymnastics which are the building the foundation for other abilities. Making sure you can perform these fundamentals flawlessly will help you to advance and enhance your gymnastics!

1. Handstand

Handstands are arguably the single most essential technique and position to be found in the gymnastics sport. Handstands are the foundation of the essential abilities required for all four of the events. The ability to perform the perfect handstand is a thing you need to learn and master. Handstands are utilized for a lot of tumbling techniques -such as handsprings and walkovers. Handstands are crucial for bars. Cast on handstands, and giants can be performed at handstands. Handsprings in vault traverse through the handstand posture. One of the key factors to mastering your back roll during the floor routine at level 6 is achieving a flawless handstand right in the middle in the rolling. Handstands can be practiced at home, by performing Spiderman on the walls. This is among my most favorite exercises to improve the gymnastics abilities at your home. Spiderman against the wall can be described as essentially doing a handstand on the wall. However, it's an exercise to improve handstapping with proper form. For Spiderman on the wall sit with your back to the wall of your home. Place your feet on the ground your face, then each time, place your feet against the wall. Bring your hands closer to the wall while you move your legs up to the wall until your stomach touches the wall, and you're in a handstand. Your feet's uppers are to be level against the wall. With your toes pointed towards the wall (your toes will be in contact with walls). Make sure your head is not tilted, and keep your hands in view with your eyes. Do this at least a few minutes before lowering your feet. When you're in the handstand, focus in tightening your muscles. Think about lifting your feet to the ceiling. It is a fantastic opportunity to perfect your posture since the wall will force your body to remain in a straight line.

2. Cast

Casting is one of the fundamental bar component, and knowing the art of casting at an early stage will enable you to acquire a myriad of other techniques. Position of the body in a cast has a hollow body form. The hollow shape of the body looks like the one you get for a perfectly upright handstand apart from the aspect that your back is slightly round and your stomach is pulled toward your spine. The goal is eventually to cast for a handstand. The more you are able to cast higher by maintaining a good, tight physique, the greater the chance of success. It is important that your legs be straight and together with your stomach tucked in while your back is rounded with your eyes focusing on the bar.

3. Splits

The ability to master side and middle splits can help you master other moves that utilize the same form as well. Your splits are also easy to learn at your home. A split "shape" is everywhere in gymnastics such as split leaps, switches, jumps, within backwalkovers and more. The more proficient you can perform your splits in the ground and the more you'll have the ability to execute these in the middle of your skill. It is recommended that you make a split using your left leg, right foot, and your middle split while keeping your legs straight until you are on the ground.

4. Handspring on Vault

Handsprings on vaults are the foundational skill vaults at the upper levels are built on. It's difficult to do well in Yurchenkos or the twisting vaults if your haven't discovered the mechanics behind handspring vault. In order to do an excellent handspring in vault, you must to sprint fast, leap at a high "punch" off the spring board, fly into the air, and then do an ideal handstand from the high on the table of vaults and then block your shoulders away from the vault's top and then land on your feet. One of the most fundamental gymnastics skills is also in play -the handstand.

5. Back Handspring

Back handsprings are an essential gymnastics skill to learn because it's the fundamental technique used for back tumbling on the floor as well as beam. It's difficult to link the higher-level skills (like designs, full twists double backs, and back tucks) with a roundoff handspring if you aren't able to do the correct back handspring. The roundoff as well as the back handspring both are crucial to provide power to anything that follows it.

6. Round-off

Roundoffs are just the same as a back handspring master for the tumbling of floors. Roundoffs provide power as the back handspring gives power for the tumbling pass.

7. Turn on 1 Foot

Turning 1 foot is a technique that will never disappear. It's a requirement in all routine of floor and beam gymnastics class 4-10. It is therefore advisable to be able to master this gymnastics fundamental skill as soon as possible.

8. Split Leap

A split jump is a different ability that is needed in each beam and floor routine stages 4-10. For a flawless split leap, you need to achieve the perfect split in the air at the highest level possible above the ground. Additionally, you should need your split to be equally as both legs need to have the same distance to the ground.

Chapter 4: Understanding Xcel And Jo Gymnastics Programs

USA Gymnastics, the largest regulator of gymnastics has provided a classic Junior Olympic (JO) level program in which gymnasts participate. When a gymnast has become competent at their level and has a score that is qualifying then he/she can choose to advance to the next stage. Levels 3-10 are competitive at the top, and once you reach level 10, a gymnast can become "elite" (those are the gymnasts who compete at an Olympics). A flaw was found in the JO levels system. For JO there's one specific mold the gymnast must meet. Gymnasts who do not meet the mold, because of physical or financial limitations the ability or commitment degree, there was no alternative but to go through the JO process. In 2013 USAG introduced an Xcel program. Xcel program. USAG describes it as Xcel programme as "a broad-based, affordable competitive experience outside of the traditional Jr. Olympic Program." Xcel is, just like JO offers several levels (Bronze silver, gold Platinum, Diamond) which gymnasts can move up to while learning new abilities. The gymnasts that participate in Xcel are also able to enjoy the competition experience as being part of an athletic team and performing before a judge.

The main major difference in JO the JO and Xcel is that while JO is very rigid in its standards, Xcel's requirements are more relaxed, and offer the gymnast to use a greater choice of techniques in addition to greater flexibility to develop and improve according to their own speed. Some gyms do not offer Xcel as well as Junior Olympic (JO) training as well as competitions. The gymnasts who might be not old enough to follow to the conventional JO pathway can benefit from Xcel which allows them to remain in training as well as compete, improve, and advance. The majority of gymnasts participating within the Xcel program participate in less competitions as JO gymnasts do in addition, it's much less costly and requires a lower time commitment as that of JO.

Xcel could be an excellent choice for young gymnasts who just wants to master the beam or the bar since in the Xcel program, they are free to train and compete in only those two areas, for what she's interested in doing. This is also an option when a gymnast is having difficulty learning an event because they won't be hindered due to the competition.

Approximate Comparison of Skill Level:

Xcel Bronze = Jo Level 3 or less Xcel Silver = Jo Level 3/4 Xcel Gold = Jo Level 5/5 Xcel Platinum = JOL Level 6/7 Xcel Diamond = JO Level 7/8and above

The JO athlete should demonstrate a an excellent level of physical fitness (including development of skills as well as strength and flexibility) in all four sports and must have a strong work ethic as well as ability to coach. The JO athlete will spend more time training in the gym and competes in more events that necessitate travel, and could be more expensive to purchase uniforms. This means that JO can be family-oriented commitment in terms of as money and time. This program is ideal for those who just would like to play gymnastics! The Xcel athlete should also show the physical capability to work hard, as well as ability to coach member of a team that competes however, without the requirements and requirements that JO has. The Xcel athlete is able to train less at the gym, and can participate in less competitions. This Xcel program is ideal for those who have potential in gymnastics, but also wishes to take on other activities or sports and for families who isn't able to financially commit to join JO.

The JO gymnastics training program is broken into 10 levels prior to you can reach the elite levels. The 10 levels align perfectly with the various levels athletes compete at as defined by USA Gymnastics - which is the body that oversees official gymnastics across the U.S. as well as named the USAG.

For you to be eligible to move into the next level, there are specific requirements are required to prove that you have learned all that you need to have learnt in the four contests at the end of last stage. One of them is to score a particular amount for a particular competition at the same level as you're in and another of the requirements is to attain a certain level of level of age.

The initial 3 levels of this program concentrate on teaching the basic principles of gymnastics. They do not require gymnasts to participate in competitions of any kind. At times, different gyms meet to organize games, fun and practice in order to get the gymnasts comfortable competing, however this is not necessary and some gyms don't conduct this in any way.

Levels 4 and 5 of Levels 4 and 5 of the JO program are referred to as the "compulsory" levels. Level 4 is the level where gymnasts compete for the first time in matches, also known as meets. At these levels, nevertheless, the routines have been set out. That means all the gymnasts are performing the exact same routines using the exact same routines all the time that they're performing these levels. Similar routines that are compulsory for all levels are performed in simplified forms in the competitions at level 3 in the event they take place.

Levels 6-10 within levels 6-10 of the JO program are known as "optional" levels. It doesn't mean you are able to choose to participate in competitions however, it means that during these levels you can begin creating your own routines, instead of having a routine you must complete. The routines you choose to do will still need certain aspects to be included in each competition, however these elements are flexible enough to work in any place in any routine the gymnast decides to place them in.

Chapter 5: Elite Gymnastics

If you've watched gymnasts compete at the Olympics and you've had aspirations of competing at an highest levels. To become an elite gymnast is not easy, but you are able to succeed if you're willing to invest the time and commitment to master the fundamental skills, and then move higher in the levels.

Gymnasts who are elite must dedicate a significant amount of time to training in order to remain fit and maintain their abilities. The exact amount of hours that you'll be required to dedicate for training isn't set as a set number, many athletes train around 30 hours a week.

After you've completed the level 10 of the Junior Olympics program, you are able to begin practicing as in the top gymnast class.

"Elite" is the highest level you could achieve within an JO class. Gymnasts in Level 10 are thought of as "Pre-Elite."

Different forms of training programs for instance, those offered by the USA Gymnastics Xcel program, is designed to assist to develop similar skills. The Xcel program is not designed to provide gymnastics training at the highest levels. [17]

Take part in a elite qualification event.

If you are able to master the Pre-Elite ability set After that, you are able to apply in The Elite Program.

Begin working with your coach to get ready for qualifying contests. They will comprise compulsory as well as optional practices.

The exact scores that you'll have to attain in each event that qualifies will vary based on your age and the types of events that you are eligible to participate in.

*You must be 11-15 years old in order to be an Junior Elite gymnast, and the age of 16 or over to be an Senior Elite gymnast.

If you're an Elite gymnast, you can become eligible for the National Team and participate in international gymnastics competitions.

Here's a quick outline of the steps to getting to be an Elite gymnast in the United States.

Gymnasts for women get to the Elite grade through a successful completion of two steps. (Note that the total points given below are up-to date from the start of 2017 and reflect the reduction of elements points that are required to be in force for 2017-20 Code of Points. Minimum scores for qualifying are susceptible to change.)

Step 1: Compulsories

Compulsories show fundamentals. Here are, for instance, the 2014 National Junior Champion Jazmyn Foberg's mandatory routines from 2013. To be able to complete the compulsory stage, the gymnast needs to earn at least 35.00 points for all 4 activities during an Regional or National Qualifying competition.

The seniors (gymnasts who turn 16 or over during the calendar year) are able to choose being able to compete in 2 or 3 events, rather than all four. If they choose to do so, gymnasts are only able to compete in the two or three events, and not on the all-around competition for that elite year provided they have passed. If you are competing in a 3-event or 2-event specialization, gymnasts need to achieve minimum scores of 17.50 in 2 events, or 26.25 for three events.

The most recent requirements for required routines can be found through the USA Gymnastics website.

Step 2: Optionals

The optional routines show off of a gymnast's individual abilities and level of skill. These are routines that can be seen in the top events. As an example this is Jazmyn performing her beam routine that she performed at the National Qualifier in 2013.

For juniors (ages 11-15) For Juniors (ages 11-15), the minimum required score for all four events is 50.00 (to be considered an Elite or to qualify for Classics). Be aware that in 2017 because of the change in required element points the required element points will be changed. A Junior gymnast will automatically be qualified to Classics when she scores 52.00 or more at the the 2016 Nationals.

To qualify to Nationals, Juniors must:

Win 50.50 or more Classics

Hit the 50.50 threshold at the end of a Team Training Camp

Finish an assignment abroad prior to the year's Nationals.

For seniors, the four-event minimum score required to qualify for Classics is at present 51.00 (a 53.00 or greater at the time of the 2016 Nationals is acceptable in the event that the gymnast participated there).

The gymnasts who compete in three events need to score at minimum 39.00 and two-event gymnasts need to be able to score at minimum 26.50 in their competitions to be eligible to Classics.

In order to qualify for Nationals the seniors need to achieve these minimum scores:

52.00 or greater for 4 events (only automatically qualified athletes to Nationals since 2016 will be Olympic team members as well as alternates)

39.75 or greater for three races (41.25 or more for eligible scores in 2016)

27.00 or more for two or more events (28.00 or greater for scores that are eligible in 2016)

How Senior Elites can earn the required score to be eligible to be eligible for the optional tests:

National Qualifiers

Team Training Camps

A member or an alternate of an international team of competition since the last season's Nationals (such as World Championships, Olympics, Jesolo, etc.)

Acquired an international contract from the year before's Nationals (e.g. a World Cup, etc.)

Any routines count toward the qualification score can be full-length routines performed on a competition surface. There are no mats placed over pits made of foam, or TumblTrak confirmation is permitted.

In addition after a gymnast performed at Classics and won, they not be required to achieve the required score each year.

Returning to level 10 after Elite

When a gymnast becomes an Elite level gymnast, she can't be able to go back to J.O. Level on the spur of the moment.

For the purpose of returning to back to the J.O. degree after Elite status has been reached, the gymnast will need apply to be dropped back into the J.O. program. This can be done by sending an "reason for change" letter by their coach, to the National Junior Olympic Committee for examination.

After reviewing Following the review, the Committee Chairman informs the coach if the request was approved or rejected. The appropriate State as well as Regional Administrative Committee Chairmen and the Regional Technical Committee Chairman are informed of the outcome.

If the application for a transfer back to J.O. was approved and the gymnast was accepted, she cannot be allowed to re-enter the elite/pre-elite program in the Elite season (through Championships of the year where she is competing at level 10.).

Pro Tip

Note: Being chosen to compete in TOPS or Hopes won't result in you being an elite gymnast. However, these programs provide fantastic stepping stone for those who have a passion and are looking to achieve elite status.

Did you even know? Fun Gymnastics Facts:

In a few instances in the history of sport there have been female and male gymnasts were able to achieve a 10/10 in which the technical panel that rated them had no reason to subtract one point off their total. The gymnasts who have achieved this comprise:

1. Nadia Comaneci, who scored seven perfect 10s during the 1976 Olympic Games in Montreal.

2. Nadia Copmaneci again scores two perfect 10s during the 1980 Games in Moscow.

3. Li Ning, who scored five perfect 10s during the 1984 Games in Los Angeles.

4. Julianne McNamara who had five perfect tens during the 1984 Olympics in Los Angeles in 1984.

Chapter 6: Gymnastics Scoring Jo, College, Elite And Olympic

Are you curious about the reason gymnasts get the scores she receives? Are you wondering how much deduction there is on a missed step, a handstand, or bent legs? If so, here's an answer for you. We must first crawl first before we are able to be able to run or walk by reviewing the J.O. program prior to moving on to typical deductions and the values that are used within the NCAA.

Junior Olympic Program (Levels 4-10)

Most gymnasts who compete across the country are part of the USA Gymnastics or J.O. program prior to going on to the elite gymnastics program or college. The J.O. Program includes levels 4-10 (with 10-being the most advanced stage) The levels are evaluated using the J.O. Code of Points. USA Gymnastics updates the code every four years, to allow the sport to to develop and grow.

The difficulty is the sole major differentiator between the various levels. In this case, achieving the prerequisites at level 10 requires with more complex skills and connections as opposed to level 9. The requirements for difficulty are clearly stated within the Code of Points to maintain the integrity of each stage and ensure that they are able to move up levels.

The majority of gymnasts get to level 10, prior to advancing to college or elite gymnastics. Level 10: Meeting the basic requirements for difficulty means that an athlete's routine will begin at 9.500. To start at a 10.0--which is desirable (more of a buffer for deductions)--gymnasts need to compete with high-difficulty skills and connections to earn "bonus points."

In order to keep the discussion on the level of a beginner We won't get into detail about the details of the bonus system. But you should be aware that an athlete's score may be fakely low due to the fact that the gymnast didn't make bonuses or hampered skills.

There are numerous possible deductions at any time however, here are a few of the most popular ones that you'll come across.

Execution flawDeduction

Flexible feet (each time).05

The legs of Bent up to 0.3

Twist the legs while crossing them. 0.10

Knee or leg separation (any event)Up To 0.2

Insufficient split (leaps and leaps that are under the 180 degrees of split) up to 0.3

The beam can wobble up to 0.3

(any event) 0.5 (any kind of) 0.5

Small hop when landing 0.10

Steps to landing0.10 per step

Out of bounds.

There's also a range of less subjective deductions judges are able to make. They can be ruled out as "insufficient sureness of performance throughout the exercise on beam" (up to 0.2 10th deduction) as well as "quality of movement to reflect personal style on floor" (up to 0.3 10th deduction). The penalties are what can make J.O. scoring difficult to determine even for skilled gymnastics fanatics.

For meets in the regular season Two judges are required to score each routine. Each judge is responsible for scoring the program, and the gymnast's final score is the total of the two scores. If the judges ' readings are less than three tenths in the initial score the judges are expected to discuss with one another in order in order to find a solution to bring their scores closer together within this area.

The event of J.O., the average score of any competition is about 8.500. The majority of gymnasts aim to achieve a minimum of 9.000

for each event that they compete in, and those who score 9.500 or higher will usually be able to get a place on the podium.

NCAA Gymnastics (Divisions I, II and III)

The three divisions are available within gymnastics in colleges. The main difference in the three divisions is how many of scholarships that a school is able to offer its gymnasts. DI programs offer the greatest athletic assistance (with the exemption from Ivy League schools and service academy, that are DI but they also have individual scholarship rules). DII teams provide around 50 percent of the scholarship opportunities offered by DI teams offer, while DIII teams are not able to provide any athletic scholarships.

Gymnasts in all three divisions score with J.O. level 10 regulations, which are accompanied by NCAA "Rules Modifications." The Rules Modifications eliminate many of the redundant Level 10 rules (like the beam's sureness) which effectively reduces the lens that scores to concentrate on a lesser amount of derogations.

The narrowing of the focus, along together with the knowledge that a majority of gymnasts making it on the elite DI teams are and clean is why scores for NCAA gymnastics tend to be more impressive than those in J.O. There are even a few of 10s that are perfect, that are almost unheard of in J.O. gymnastics.

For example, form breaks such as the flex of feet, legs that are separated and bent knees can be considered to be a factor in college, but. Below are some other focus points in NCAA scoring.

What to do (no deduction)What NOT to Do (points earned)

Floor landing must end with a controlled lunges or stickUncontrolled step or jump

Bar, vault, beam landingMust be stuckStep

Bars must be with handstands at least 10 degrees vertical and less than 10 degrees away from the vertical

The vault table must be amplitude-adjusted. All turns and turning is required to be performed by putting your chest at a minimum the table. There is no an amplitude from the table

Floor and beams must be higher than 180 degrees

No balance checkBalance on beam. balance

FloorLanding with amplitude and rotation by bringing your chest upwards, and landing with your chest down

The Start Value is a different way the gymnast in college can be sacked of points. Because NCAA gymnastics is built on levels 10 and routines begin at 9.500 and gymnasts are required to complete five tenths worth of additional skills in order in order to maximise their scoring.

Start values are significant for NCAA gymnastics because the gaps between scores diminish. Gymnasts who are on elite five teams have 9.900 or greater on virtually every count routine. the distinction between an 9.950 start score or one with a 10.0 starting value can be the difference between winning and winning at a championship event.

Though the majority of JO gymnasts play with their other athletes, it's primarily one-on-one sport. NCAA gymnastics on the contrary is a truly team sport. That's the reason it is loved by numerous people, and it is thrilling and enjoyable to witness. Positive attitude and school spirit are vital components of college gymnastics.

What happens: Six gymnasts participate on every equipment and 5 scores count which means teams have to lower their lowest scores on each of the events. The five scores combined to form the team's total event score which is then the 4 event scores add to create a team's total score. The maximum score the team is likely to achieve is 200. Most often, we find the best DI teams within the 197-198 age band.

The problem is that these scores don't translate across the three divisions. Since DI teams provide the most athletic support in comparison to DII or DIII programs, it is not uncommon to find top talent gravitating to these programs. There is also some disagreement regarding how scores are given to routines in DII and, more specifically, DIII, with certain observers insisting that the judges grade the routines similar to J.O. Level 10--without any changes.

Elite & Olympic Scoring

It is here that things begin to become bizarre.

At the level of 10, skilled gymnasts may be able to enter the U.S. Elite program. There, they'll get the chance to compete for this country and the United States at international competitions. The gymnasts who are selected for this program are among the elite in

America and typically skip regular classes in order to work full-time. In the gymnasts who are there, only few will possess the ability to make it onto the Olympic team.

For the elite programs There isn't a anything as a perfect 10. In 2006, the International Gymnastics Federation (FIG)--the worldwide governing body for competitive gymnastics--implemented a new system of scoring to encourage and reward gymnasts for competing difficult routines.

The final score the gymnast earns at any occasion is the result of two distinct elements. The first is The Difficulty ("D") score which comprises connection values and the difficulty of skill. Another is The Execution ("E") score and is comparable with the J.O. system, in that the score begins at 10 and goes down as penalty points are taken.

But, the FIG Code is a lot rougher than J.O. Code, with the E Score. As an example, a drop in J.O. is counted as a deduction of five-tenths however a drop in FIG constitutes a full point.

In contrast to NCAA athletes, gymnasts of elite level can't make controlled leaps out of their tumbling moves. They must stay with every move. One technique that elite gymnasts employ to manage their passes and reduce deductions is to jump or leap from their tumble (it's much easier to master a jump as it is to manage the double twisting of a double salto).

The D Score functions as the start-value in that the gymnast gets rewarded for executing challenging skills and combination. Instead of seeking to narrow the gap that exists between a minimum beginning value and 10.0 score, the D Score isn't determined by a maximum threshold. The harder an athlete has in performing her best and competitive competition, the greater the D Score.

If Olympians in beam meet the three or four techniques within a row and do so, they are awarded a higher D Score when they do this. If a gymnast is required to link a sequence of abilities but stumbles between, she will break the link and loses difficulties points. In floor gymnastics, the best athletes make four tumble passes instead of three in order maximise the chance to master difficult techniques.

Simone Biles is the best gymnast on the planet principally due to her score on the D. Biles is a tonne of challenges in each event. So absurd, in fact that she can be thrown down multiple times (incurring an entire point each time) but still be able to win due to the D Score she scores is highly competitive. Also, she's extremely clean in each event, which means that her E Score is lethal as is her E Score as well. Add them all together and you've got an invincible rival.

In all-around qualifying for at the 2018. World Championships, for example, Simone won the competition with a near 4 points lead. In vault and floor, her two most successful events, Simone had scores that was 6.4 and 6.7 and 6.7, respectively. The second-place winner, Morgan Hurd tallied a 5.4 and 5.5 in these two events. The point score in gymnastics is substantial, and allows Simone the opportunity to make mistakes and be able to win.

The top finishers in the Olympics generally get a score of 15.000 or more in the day, whereas those at lower levels of the podium could instead strive at a number within the mid-14.0 band. For the most elite international competitions those who score a score of 13 or less won't be considered competitive.

For putting the standard of elite gymnastics in perspective Even competitors with lower scores are highly sought-after by elite NCAA teams. Due to the elite programs' rigorous standards in terms of fitness and technique and form, anyone who has the abilities to move to elite level will become a star athlete in the college. If you're one of the elite gymnasts and believe that their journey has completed through the mud, NCAA gymnastics is a area where they will find new success, and also be having fun.

Men's Artistic Scoring

The scoring of International/Elite, Junior Olympics and Future Stars can be found below.

Elite/International Scoring

It is the International Gymnastics Federation's (FIG) score system, which is used for female and male gymnastics, established in January 2006 and updated to the 2009-2012 quadrennial, includes credits for routine's quality as well as its difficulty, execution and content, and also for the artistry of the female athletes. For the United States, this system is in use at all of the top levels of competition. Ladies' Junior Olympics (Levels 1-10) and gymnastics at collegiate level employ the system built on an 10.0 maximal score, while male Junior Olympics and collegiate gymnastics utilize a modified version of FIG. FIG scoring method.

Additionally to the scoring process, FIG's scoring process is guided with the Code of

Points, which changes for each quadrennial period by revising the abilities of players and changing individual apparatus needs. The 2006 system which removed the requirement for the 10 point maximum was adopted at a meeting at Baku, Azerbaijan, in October 2005. The system has since been updated for the 2009-12 quadrennium. The basic procedure is identical for both females and males, a few variations exist between the two. Both the men's and women's scoring system is like the ones used for the rhythmic gymnastics, trampoline tossing, as well as in acrobatic gymnastics.

According to the current model, a gymnast's complete score is comprised of the entire routine's content as well as the ability to execute. Basically, the scoring procedure adds the Difficulty Score, which includes difficulty value for skills, connection value and element/compositional requirements, to the Execution Score, which encompasses execution - and for women, artistry on the balance beam and floor exercise - to determine a gymnast's total score. Scores are no longer able to have the maximum of 10.

Difficulty Score: difficult as well as technical content. This score (previously known as the starting value) comprises credit for the number of specific skills that are performed during the exercise and also connect value (credit for linking high-level competencies) as well as compositional or element group demands. Men make use of the word element group requirements. These constitute the fundamental types of competencies or elements that need to be included in routines. Women use composition rather than element group in order to define this need. Compositional or element requirements are different according to the apparatus. This score is derived through the D (Difficulty) Panel that is a two-person panel.

The amount of difficulty is calculated through the totalization of values for the hardest skills, which are eight for women and ten for men, which include the ability to dismount. Every skill is assigned a level of difficulty, which is defined within the Code of Points, and can be classified into seven categories. The value for difficulty of an element or skill will not be acknowledged in the event that it is not able to satisfy the requirements of its technology. Additionally, credits are only granted once per ability. The women have to perform at least three dance components as well as a maximum of five Acrobatics in their floor and balance beam routines.

Connection values are awarded after particular skills or kinds of abilities can be successfully executed at a consistent pace. The females can earn connections values by performing the bar with the balance beam or uneven bars as well as the floor exercises, while males can get it from the exercise on the floor and for the horizontal bar. The same applies to women and men. the connection value for each is 0.1 or 0.2 points. The connection value will not be awarded in the event that a gymnast falls.

Compositional and element group requirements comprise the fundamental skills or components which must be in every program and are different for each the equipment. The requirements in this area are similar to those special requirements that were in place that were previously required. When all five requirements are met the maximum amount of 2.5 points will be given.

Each member of the D Panel independently reaches his/her Difficulty Score. The two judges compare their scores and come to the same consensus.

Once the score is recorded, a coach could seek clarification on the difficulty score initially verbally, and later in writing. A question can be answered through video review. An initial inquiry should be filed prior to end of the gymnast's exercise. Written inquiries is due prior to the time of the turn before it is then that the Superior Jury reviews the inquiry. When attending FIG occasions the fee will be assessed for submitting an inquiry. it's returned when an inquiry is accepted.

Execution Score: performance, and for women, art (balance beam and floor exercises). The Execution Score is determined by six members of the E Panel, now begins at 10 and deducts are taken for mishaps and errors with regard to technique, execution and art. Each judge decides independently on the score of his/her judge. Scores that are lowest and highest are eliminated, while Gymnasts' Execution Score becomes the total of the other four judges score. Negative errors that are deducted for are deducted from the total of the Execution and Difficulty Scores.

The deductibility for different errors vary between 0.1 point for a minor mistake to 1.00 points for falling. Negative deductions are for breaking the rules or not complying with time limits and also for attire or podium violation.

The right to inquire is not available on execution Score.

Score total. The gymnast's final score will be that of the Total score for Difficulty and Execution plus any deductions made for non-neutral errors. Here's an example of how scoring is determined. The sample uses the routine of a woman.

Bars with uneven surfaces

Complexity (4C=4x0.3, 4D=4x0.4)+2.8 points

Element groups (5x0.5) +2.5 points

Connect value = +0.6 points

TDS Score 5.9 points

Execution Score*

Start of the base 10 points

Deductions and Execution -0.7 points

Artistry -0.3 points

Overall execution score 9.0 points

Score at the end 14.9 points

Note: In the case of the floor and balance beam exercises, the program's breakdown might include one acrobatic skill of E-level and 2 D-level acrobatic abilities and 2 C-level acrobatic abilities and 2 dance moves of C-level and one B-level dance movement. A gymnast can add more dance components if they're more valuable than Acrobatic moves. But, the total amount of dance elements can not be more than eight. The value of the dismount is always considered, regardless of its significance.

*The Execution Score is determined using averaging of the middle four scores of the six.

Also, for males deductions are listed under workout presentation deductions, rather than separated into artistry and execution.

The number of connections that is used in this example is just for women, and is not an appropriate number for males.

This is a description of the setup during FIG events like events like the Olympic Games,

World Championships and World Cups. The members of the two panels can differ at other events not run by FIG. FIG. The scoring process and the scoring system remain the same, although the amount of judges for the panels could change.

If the system is utilized it is possible that the FIG can make changes when needed. This was done previously with various adjustments. While there is no longer a "10" designation is no not the highest score anymore however, the new system allows viewers to know how a gymnast scored and the method of determining it. The present method is a fresh calculation of earlier pieces of starting values, deducts, and scores.

Scoring Example

Below is a score comparison between the current scoring system as well as the previous system that utilized the 10 points maximum. It was based on the balance beam routine performed by Carly Patterson that was used in the finals of the 2004 Olympic Games. This was intended solely as a visual aid to illustrate the distinctions between the two scoring systems. Be aware that this program was developed under the older system. Routines that use using the current code will not be built this way. This is meant to be used as a framework of reference. The 2004 Olympic Games, Patterson's routine was scored 9.775 from 10.0.

Details about the scoring systemNew score systemOld scoring system

Breakdown of routine

Mount: Split sitNo ValueA

Standing scale split No ValueA

Standing Arabian saltoFE (0.2)

Front aerial, flic flac reverse layout, step outD B C (Acrobatic Series) +0.20 Connection value: D+B+C (0.2) + (0.1)

Front salto, sheep jump D, D +0.10 Connection value D+D (0.2) + (0.2)

Half turnNo ValueNo Value

Full turn AA

Jump switch, back tuck C, C +0.10 Connection C+C (0.1)

Dismount: Round-off. Flic flac 2 feet, two Arabian saltoB, B G +0.20 Connection value B+B+SuperE (0.2)+ (0.2)

Total Bonus 1.4

Routine evaluation to calculate Difficulty ScoreUnder the current system, the elements that count difficulty include:

The basic starting value is 8.8

1. Acrobatic G equals 0.7

1 Acrobatic F = 0.6

2 D. acrobatic = 0.8

1 Acrobatic C is 0.3

1 D dance = 0.4 1 C dance = 0.3 1 A dance = 0.1

Difficulty score, 3.2

The dance routine will be awarded 2.0 from a possible 2.5 in compositional demands (CR) due to the fact that there's the dance routine is not composed of 2 elements with 180 crosses splits. Split Routines begin with 8.8 base and add 1.4 bonus. The the maximum starting value of 10.0

CR, 2.0

Connection bonus 0.6

0.1 for front saltos to jump sheep

0.1 for a switch jump to reverse salto

0.2 for front aerials Flic flac, layout salto

0.2 to round-off and flic flac. Double Arabian dismount

The Difficulty Score/start value TOTAL Difficulty score: 5.810.0 SV

E Panel Deductions

Nomount of value Composition deduction 0.1

Execution deduction, 0.3

Take the 0.1 compositional as well as the 0.3 execution deductions. Subtract from 10.0

Execution Score/ Deductions TOTAL Execution Score 9.6Execution Deductions 0.25

Deductions and explanations for executions Assuming that judges take (2) -0.1 deductions as well as (1) -0.05 deduction, and realizing that execution penalty are no longer the 0.05 deduction The minimum deduction required of execution is now 0.3. The absence of a dance routine and there is no mount for the element

Final Score(Difficulty as well as the Execution Scores) 15.49.775

FIG Scoring System Comparison

Note: This description of the scoring system currently in use is based on the structure used at FIG events, such as events like the Olympic Games, World Championships and World Cups. The size of the two juries might differ at other events that are not controlled by FIG. FIG. The scoring process and the scoring system are the same throughout, however the number of judges on juries can alter. When the system is being utilized and the FIG could make changes according to the need, as is what has happened previously with different modifications.

The current systemOld version, 10 points. maximum scoring system

Each gymnast's ScoreScore is calculated by adding the score of the content of the routine (Difficulty Score) and its execution (Execution Score). Each exercise was assigned a starting value, while it was the sum of credits awarded for the exercise, less deductions based on the execution. The best score that could be achieved for each routine was calculated by the starting value. There was a the maximum score being 10 points.

Start value/D ScoreIs now part of the score determined by D Panel, which includes difficulty value, compositional/element group requirements (which vary by apparatus) and connection value. Men refer to the requirements for skill as "element group requirements" and the females are referring to it as "compositional requirements." Start values were determined by the specific elements that were that were included in the program and also the added value to connections, as well as any other bonus elements. Starting point at the level of elite was 8.8 for females and 8.4 for males. The highest was 10.

D Panel The two-person panel which determines the Difficulty Score as well as the highest difficulty and the value of content of every routine. Only judges of the highest standard are eligible to participate in this panel.The two-person panel decided the starting value for each program. Only judges of the highest rank were eligible and usually comprised people from the technical committee. It was referred to as Jury A.

E Pane consists of six judges. E Panel evaluates routines for the execution, technicality and especially for females, talent. Every judge begins by assessing 10 before making deductions for errors committed within those categories. This is the size of the panel at FIG-organized international events. the size may differ for national events.Made with Six judges Jury B evaluated a program based on its performance, technique, and artistic. Jury B worked very similarly as Jury A, which was similar to the E Panel but did not begin at a point of 10 to determine score. Instead, it added up the scores and deductions. The judge with the lowest and highest scored were discarded while the other four scores were summed, then subtracting the starting value, resulting in the gymnast's total score. The highest attainable score for a routine was determined by the start value; the maximum available was 10.Difficulty (D) Score: difficulty and technical content scoreThe Difficulty Score includes points for difficulty value, compositional/element group requirements and connection value. D Panel determines this for every exercise. The score is basically an equivalent to the starting value. Men was the largest portion of the scores and was known as the score of difficulty. The score was derived by an An panel.

Value of difficulty (part of the Difficulty Score)Points are awarded to those elements that are ranked the best 10. For men, 10 and eight for females, with the exception of dismount. In order to be able to perform the balance beam or floor exercises, females must be able to perform at least three dances with up to five acrobatic moves during their routine. The degree of difficulty of an element will not be recognized when it does not meet the technical requirements. Skills are classified into seven categories, A to G. The value of difficulty is an element of the Difficulty score. Point values for the skills and categories have been updated. The starting value comprised the base score and bonus points, which were derived through connections and the values. For men, this was known as the difficulty score, and it was divided into Difficulty and Bonus Points. Women and men's abilities were classified into six different groups of difficultness, ranging from A to Super E.

Value of connection (part of the Difficulty Score)Included within the score. Connection value can be earned by men during two of six activities (floor and horizontal bars) while women can have it when they do in three of the four (beam flooring, floor, uneven bars, beam). The credit is granted only when the skill is performed with no fall or any other requirements. Connections are valued at 0.1 and 0.2 points. This was included in the beginning value. Connection values were recorded for men at five occasions, while the females had three. The credit was given only for skills that were executed without falling, or for women, when they had more then 0.3 per deduction.

Compositional/Element Group Requirement (part of Difficulty Score) The women call this requirement "composition" and the men use the phrase "element group." Each apparatus has five identified compositional/element groups and each of the five element groups is awarded 0.5 pts, with a maximum of 2.5 available. The same is not the case for vaults. The requirement was for the starting value of. The men's code is similar to the 2001-05 Code, with the difference that every element group had a value of 0.1.

Execution Score: Performance, art, E Panel, gymnasts are given a score on the basis of the technique, execution and, for women the artistry (balance beam and floor exercises). Scores begin at 10 and then deductions are awarded for mistakes in the execution or artistic performance. The judges with the highest and lowest score are eliminated. Four judges' scores are then taken into account as averages.

Chapter 7: The Difference Between Usag And Aau

USA Gymnastics, also referred to as USAG is a United States-based sport organization at the national level which culminates with the U.S. Olympic team one. It is also known as the AAU can be described as a league comprising a number of clubs and teams who play each other out for team and individual competitions. The two organizations provide gymnastics opportunities both for boys and girls.

USA Gymnastics, also referred to as USAG is a national sport organization which culminates with the U.S. Olympic team.

The AAU is a league comprised of a variety of teams and clubs that play each other out both in team and individual events. Both clubs offer gymnastics programs both for boys and girls. USAG has more stringent rules and more specialized on competition levels, specifically created to provide athletes with the best nutrition.

Amateur Competition

AAU means Amateur Athletic Union, and AAU gymnasts cannot perform at a professional level. This eliminates the possibility of receiving the possibility of financial compensation or other professional advantages to the gymnasts. USA Gymnastics offers professional memberships for judges, coaches and competitive coaches and meet directors who are qualified. The majority of staff and coaches who assist in helping in the running of AAU events are the parents of the kids participating in events and games. Both AAU as well as the USAG are non-profit organizations.

Benefits

Both AAU as well as USAG need athletes to be the appropriate memberships to be able to participate in their respective sports However, the benefits of membership between the two organisations are different. The USAG gives gymnasts discounts on clothing along with an AAU membership card and decal. AAU members enjoy discounts at Enterprise Rent-A-Car, Motel 6 as well as other companies that are members. AAU members get different levels of insurance for competitions and during training.

Level Requirements

Both AAU as well as the USAG provide distinct levels where your child may compete according to their ability. Although the AAU suggests appropriate levels of competition for athletes, there aren't any specific requirements for eligibility or mobility for competing at a certain degree. USAG needs tryouts as well as specific contests to determine whether your child is able to move higher in rank or at a certain the level at which they compete. This is why the USAG gives more intense level of competition to highly competent gymnasts.

"Every single element, even the most hair-raising, can be improved. "Dmitry Bilozerchev. Dmitry Bilozerchev.

Chapter 8: Other Gymnastics Programs (Tops, Hopes, And Future Stars)

TOPS and HOPES comprise training programs only available to USAG that are designed specifically for younger gymnasts of females with the potential of elite athletes. The two programs are designed for kids aged 8 to. In order to be eligible the child has to pass the rigorous test conducted by USAG. These programs assess beam complexity as well as overall fitness and techniques. Training camps are provided across the United States, making it possible for both you and your child to become involved in the sport without moving further across the country. Boys, on the other hand, USAG offers similar training programs - Elite as well as Future Stars for five different levels of age.

One of the most well-known and well-known of them all are the TOPs gymnastics programme. TOPs refers to Talent Opportunity Program and has been in existence for less than 25 years. HOPES was previously named TOPs Elite and the two programs have a lot in common.

The main difference in these two programs is the fact that TOPs are performed in conjunction with regular JO levels, while HOPEs is more focused specifically on competitions it has its own as well as training sessions, offering its gymnasts the experience of what is like to attain elite levels.

These two programmes are only open to those who have been invited. At times, it is the case that there is the help of a talent scout. However, in other instances, the coach of gymnastics can recognize the talent of their own child. In either case, after the gymnast is noticed, the next thing to do is be able to pass some tests. The aim of both these programs is to find gymnasts who have the capacity to reach the elite level, and to make them successful, and so the test is extremely strict which results in not every gymnast who is identified as a candidate passes.

In this scenario most of the girls who are taking the test for TOPs have a range of 7 to 10 years old, with only a little older or younger than the age groups. The TOPs program is a regional test in July or June, and If the gymnast performs adequately, they attend the national competition during October. If they score a high enough scores there, they are then able the opportunity to attend a fitness session in the month of December.

The tests are divided according to age, with the sole requirement for the gymnasts who are 7 years old are the 6 tests of flexibility that gymnasts of all ages must complete. The first test tests is the rope climb, which is 12' tall and not making use of your legs. They have to be held in a pike in a seated position. Another test is to hold the handstand for 30 minutes while in the proper place.

The tests for the third and fourth consist of a specific number of press handstands as well as leg lifts. The fifth test will be doing some handstands that are cast onto the bar. The final test involves six holds and 6 kicks.

Each of these tests will be graded based on how the gymnast is able to complete the task and whether they maintained the correct manner of performing. Gymnasts between 8 and 10 year old are also required to take basic assessments for each of the three competitions, in addition to the vault, which they also score in.

If the gymnast is able to pass the test and begins program and is accepted into the program, they will be expected to complete many more training hours regularly, if not every day basis. Occasionally, depending on the facility the TOPs gymnasts might not compete in any way apart from when they progress to higher levels, as they're concentrating all their efforts on their exercise. Continuous training and doing absolutely nothing else could be very exhausting on gymnasts, and that is the reason why some gymnasts is able to quit the program once they have been in it for a few weeks. The HOPES program, each gymnast is evaluated every year, with athletes who didn't perform sufficiently well being kicked from the group. The reason is that the program can take too long that a lot youngsters who are interested in it, decide to attend homeschooling in order that they are able to keep up with the gymnastics instruction.

Although there is more fun but lots of work involved within TOPs, if you're willing to work hard and have fun in the TOPs program, it's the most likely way to be a pro-level gymnast. Furthermore, during 2012's Olympics all five female athletes of the Olympics Gymnastics team were part of the TOPs program. This is an additional reason it could be beneficial to look in the TOPs program if you're hoping to one day be there.

"I'd rather regret the risks that didn't work out than the chances I didn't take at all."

- Simone Bile.

Chapter 9: Collegiate Gymnastics

The sport of gymnastics is offered to women in the 81 NCAA institutions and universities, with a majority of them having Division 1 schools. Athletes who wish to participating at this level have to study the schools they are interested in, and then review the roster of athletes to comprehend the opportunities available. In this article we'll examine the differentiators between all three NCAA divisions. We also discuss the various gymnastics-related colleges, to help athletes build a an impressive list of colleges to consider.

Which colleges offer female gymnastics teams?

In terms of recruitment, gymnastics for women is among the sports that is most competitive out in the world. There are just eight gymnastics clubs across the nation, which are which are home to more than 1,000 gymnasts. The majority of them, 62 schools, compete on the Division 1 levels. Division 2 provides the least possibilities, offering only five schools. This does not mean that athletes should be ignoring this particular level. Division 2 schools provide great sporting opportunities, frequently competing with Division 1 programs in addition to athletic awards.

The Division 3 has 15 gymnastics schools for women, and although the field is small but the potential is high. The Division 3 athletes compete with Division 2 and Division 1 programs frequently. In addition, students often discover that Division 3 provides more opportunities to concentrate on their academics, take part-time jobs and even participate in work experience.

Which NCAA Division 1 Women's Gymnastics teams exist?

It is 62 division I gymnastics institutions across the United States, and competing across a range of conferences including SEC, MPSF, Pac-12, MAC, MRGC, ECAC, MIC, Big 12, EAGL and Big Ten. These conferences let athletes and teams are eligible for national championships by winning the preliminary contests in four regions. In simple terms, the challenge is quite tough. Division 1 sports is as a full-time occupation, in which athletes are required to train throughout the year. The payoff, in the end, is definitely worthwhile for athletes looking to play at the highest level possible.

Big Ten = Big Ten Conference

Big 12 = Big 12 Conference

EAGL = East Atlantic Gymnastics League

GEC = Gymnastics East Conference

Ind. = Independent

MAC - Mid-American Conferece

MPSF = Mountain Pacific Sports Federation

NCGA = National Collegiate Gymnastics Association

Pac-12 = Pacific-12 Conference

SEC = Southeastern Conference

WIAC = Wisconsin Intercollegiate Athletic Conference

How many gymnastics schools in Division 2 do you know of?

Five D2 gymnastics facilities with only five D2 gymnastics schools, Division 2 gymnastics is by far the least populated division of the NCAA. It is located throughout all of the U.S. in Connecticut, Missouri, Washington, Texas and Pennsylvania and vary in terms of study body numbers in the range of Seattle Pacific University at about 3,800 students up to West Chester University of Pennsylvania which has more than 17,000 students. The schools are part of three conference groups, which include the Midwest Independent Conference, the Mountain Pacific Sports Federation, as well as the Eastern College Athletic Conference, in addition to competing against Division 1 teams.

Achieving a scholarship in one of the Division 2 gymnastics schools is highly competitive as there are a mere 100 gymnasts with scholarships of 36 available. But, coaches are able to split the funds between gymnasts, and offer partial scholarships to a variety of athletes in their teams.

What number of Division 3 gymnastics teams do you know of across the nation?

There are an 81 NCAA women's gymnastics teams across the nation, including 15 which are part of Division 3 colleges. Over the past 10 years, two of the D3 gymnastics teams have cut their programming--MIT and Wilson College. But they still have club teams.

As the gymnastics scene in Division 3 is small students are often shocked by the fact that they often play with Division 1 and two schools. Thus with regards to ability level, there's an overlap in the gymnasts' capabilities. Apart from learning new abilities the majority of athletes opt for Division 3 gymnastics schools since it allows them to take part at multiple events.

Which colleges provide women's gymnastics scholarship?

NCAA Division 1 and Division 2 gymnastics schools can provide athletic scholarship opportunities. Only 5 Division I sports which have head count scholarships available, and women's gymnastics is among of the five. The Division 1 coaches of gymnastics may award up to 12 scholarships for head counts which are full ride scholarship. This means that coaches in this class offer all-inclusive scholarships to 12 players on their team during the academic year.

Division 2 however, offers up to six scholarship. That means coaches are provided with a pool of athletic money and can allocate this aid to any athletes they'd like however they wish. In general, coaches split the scholarships into part scholarships and provide aid to several teammates.

While Division 3 schools cannot legally provide sports scholarships, they are able to offer financial aid that consists of academic grants, scholarships based on need as well as grants. Athletes with good grades and excellent score may be able to find Division 3 schools have scholarships that are competitive compared to other schools.

Which are the top colleges for gymnastics teams?

In terms of gymnastics-related colleges, students only have a few options. There are just 89 gymnastics schools in the United States with 62 of these are Division 1 colleges, which makes the competition more challenging. Many recruits opt for these top programs once they look for a college. However, there are a variety of aspects to take into consideration when choosing which gymnastics school to go to.

Athletics certainly play an important role in college, however there are also other factors like location, academics costs, and other factors to take into consideration. Be aware that college admissions is not a one-way road in that, to really fit to the school, players must be a fan of the college just as the sports programme.

See NCSA's top list of top gymnastics schools for students athletes.

The rankings for gymnastics at the women's level

The College Gymnastics Association provides college gymnastics ranking for every NCAA teams in addition to individuals. The following are the 10 best colleges gymnastics teams according to National qualifying scores:

1. University of Michigan

2. University of Utah

3. University of Oklahoma

4. University of Florida

5. University of Denver

6. Louisiana State University

7. University of Minnesota

8. Auburn University

9. University of Alabama

10. University of Missouri

The rankings offer a glimpse of the top gymnastics schools, however the truth is that college coaches have the highest percentage of gymnasts at high school in the nation. Although athletics are a major aspect to take into account in making a college selection however, each family's personal preferences will be unique to each family.

Furthermore, if an applicant spends all their efforts into getting accepted into a school which isn't the right fit to them academically or athletically it's a missed opportunity to have great opportunities to interact with coaches from different programs. It is recommended to research different schools for the ideal match for you. A good first step is to study the gymnastics skill guidelines that provide a base on what coaches look for in each division.

Colleges which have gymnastics teams. Currently, there are gymnastics programs totalling 89 across the United States. Find the entire list of gymnastics colleges here.

Arizona State University

Tempe, Arizona

South West

Pacific-12 Conference

NCAA D1

Auburn University

Auburn, Alabama

South East

Southeastern Conference

NCAA D1

Augustana University - South Dakota

Sioux Falls, South Dakota

North West

Northern Sun Intercollegiate Conference

NCAA D2

Ball State University

Muncie, Indiana

Great Lakes

Mid-American Conference

NCAA D1

Brigham Young University

Provo, Utah

South West

West Coast Conference

NCAA D1

Boise State University

Boise, Idaho

North West

Mountain West Conference

NCAA D1

Bowling Green State University

Bowling Green, Ohio

Great Lakes

Mid-American Conference

NCAA D1

Brown University

Providence, Rhode Island

New England

Ivy League

NCAA D1

California State University - Sacramento

Sacramento, California

West Coast

Big Sky Conference

NCAA D1

Chowan University

Murfreesboro, North Carolina

Mid East

Conference Carolinas

NCAA D2

Centenary College of Louisiana

Shreveport, Louisiana

Mid South

Southern Collegiate Athletic Conference

NCAA D1

Central Michigan University

Mount Pleasant, Michigan

Great Lakes

Mid-American Conference

NCAA D1

Cornell University

Ithaca, New York

North East

Ivy League

NCAA D1

East Stroudsburg University of Pennsylvania

East Stroudsburg, Pennsylvania

North East

Pennsylvania State Athletic Conference

NCAA D2

Eastern Michigan University

Ypsilanti, Michigan

Great Lakes

Mid-American Conference

NCAA D1

George Washington University

Washington, District Of Columbia

North East

Atlantic 10 Conference

NCAA D1

Greenville University

Greenville, Illinois

Great Lakes

Upper Midwest Athletic Conference

NCAA D3

Gustavus Adolphus College

Saint Peter, Minnesota

Mid West

Minnesota Intercollegiate Athletic Conference

NCAA D3

Hamline University

Saint Paul, Minnesota

Mid West

Minnesota Intercollegiate Athletic Conference

NCAA D3

Illinois State University

Normal, Illinois

Great Lakes

Missouri Valley Conference

NCAA D1

Iowa State University

Ames, Iowa

Mid West

Big 12 Conference

NCAA D1

Ithaca College

Ithaca, New York

North East

Liberty League

NCAA D3

Kent State University

Kent, Ohio

Great Lakes

Mid-American Conference

NCAA D1

Lindenwood University

Saint Charles, Missouri

Mid West

Great Lakes Valley Conference

NCAA D2

Long Island University

Brooklyn, New York

North East

Northeast Conference

NCAA D1

Louisiana State University (LSU)

Baton Rouge, Louisiana

Mid South

Southeastern Conference

NCAA D1

Michigan State University

East Lansing, Michigan

Great Lakes

Big Ten Conference

NCAA D1

North Carolina State University

Raleigh, North Carolina

Mid East

Atlantic Coast Conference

NCAA D1

Northern Illinois University

DeKalb, Illinois

Great Lakes

Mid-American Conference

NCAA D1

Notre Dame College

Cleveland, Ohio

Great Lakes

Mountain East Conference

NCAA D2

Ohio State University

Columbus, Ohio

Great Lakes

Big Ten Conference

NCAA D1

Oregon State University

Corvallis, Oregon

West Coast

Pacific-12 Conference

NCAA D1

Penn State

University Park, Pennsylvania

North East

Big Ten Conference

NCAA D1

Rhode Island College

Providence, Rhode Island

New England

Little East Conference

NCAA D3

Rutgers University

Piscataway, New Jersey

North East

Big Ten Conference

NCAA D1

San Jose State University

San Jose, California

West Coast

Mountain West Conference

NCAA D1

Simpson College

Indianola, Iowa

Mid West

Iowa Intercollegiate Athletic Conference

NCAA D3

Southeast Missouri State University

Cape Girardeau, Missouri

Mid West

Ohio Valley Conference

NCAA D1

Southern Connecticut State University

New Haven, Connecticut

New England

Northeast-10 Conference

NCAA D2

Southern Utah University

Cedar City, Utah

South West

Big Sky Conference

NCAA D1

Springfield College

Springfield, Massachusetts

New England

National Collegiate Gymnastics Association

NCAA D3

Stanford University

Stanford, California

West Coast

Pacific-12 Conference

NCAA D1

SUNY College at Brockport

Brockport, New York

North East

Empire 8 Athletic Conference

NCAA D3

SUNY Cortland

Cortland, New York

North East

State University of New York Athletic Conference

NCAA D3

Temple University

Philadelphia, Pennsylvania

North East

American Athletic Conference

NCAA D1

Texas Woman's University

Denton, Texas

Mid South

Lone Star Conference

NCAA D2

Towson University

Towson, Maryland

North East

Colonial Athletic Association

NCAA D1

United States Air Force Academy

USAFA, Colorado

South West

Mountain West Conference

NCAA D1

University of Alabama

Tuscaloosa, Alabama

South East

Southeastern Conference

NCAA D1

University of Alaska - Anchorage

Anchorage, Alaska

West Coast

Great Northwest Athletic Conference

NCAA D1

University of California - Davis

Davis, California

West Coast

Mountain Pacific Sports Federation

NCAA D1

University of Arizona

Tucson, Arizona

South West

Pacific-12 Conference

NCAA D1

University of Arkansas

Fayetteville, Arkansas

Mid South

Southeastern Conference

NCAA D1

University of Bridgeport

Bridgeport, Connecticut

New England

East Coast Conference

NCAA D2

University of California

Berkeley, California

West Coast

Pacific-12 Conference

NCAA D1

University of California - Los Angeles - UCLA

Los Angeles, California

West Coast

Pacific-12 Conference

NCAA D1

University of Denver

Denver, Colorado

South West

Big 12 Conference

NCAA D1

University of Florida

Gainesville, Florida

South East

Southeastern Conference

NCAA D1

University of Georgia

Athens, Georgia

South East

Southeastern Conference

NCAA D1

University of Illinois

Champaign, Illinois

Great Lakes

Big Ten Conference

NCAA D1

University of Iowa

Iowa City, Iowa

Mid West

Big Ten Conference

NCAA D1

University of Kentucky

Lexington, Kentucky

Mid East

Southeastern Conference

NCAA D1

University of Maryland

College Park, Maryland

North East

Big Ten Conference

NCAA D1

University of Michigan

Ann Arbor, Michigan

Great Lakes

Big Ten Conference

NCAA D1

University of Minnesota

Minneapolis, Minnesota

Mid West

Big Ten Conference

NCAA D1

University of Missouri

Columbia, Missouri

Mid West

Southeastern Conference

NCAA D1

University of Nebraska

Lincoln, Nebraska

Mid West

Big Ten Conference

NCAA D1

University of New Hampshire

Durham, New Hampshire

New England

Eastern Atlantic Gymnastics League

NCAA D1

University of North Carolina at Chapel Hill

Chapel Hill, North Carolina

Mid East

Atlantic Coast Conference

NCAA D1

University of Oklahoma

Norman, Oklahoma

Mid South

Big 12 Conference

NCAA D1

University of Pennsylvania - Penn

Philadelphia, Pennsylvania

North East

Ivy League

NCAA D1

University of Pittsburgh

Pittsburgh, Pennsylvania

North East

Atlantic Coast Conference

NCAA D1

University of Utah

Salt Lake City, Utah

South West

Pacific-12 Conference

NCAA D1

University of Washington

Seattle, Washington

West Coast

Pacific-12 Conference

NCAA D1

University of Wisconsin - Eau Claire

Eau Claire, Wisconsin

Great Lakes

Wisconsin Intercollegiate Athletic Conference

NCAA D3

University of Wisconsin - La Crosse

La Crosse, Wisconsin

Great Lakes

Wisconsin Intercollegiate Athletic Conference

NCAA D3

University of Wisconsin - Oshkosh

Oshkosh, Wisconsin

Great Lakes

Wisconsin Intercollegiate Athletic Conference

NCAA D3

University of Wisconsin - Stout

Menomonie, Wisconsin

Great Lakes

Wisconsin Intercollegiate Athletic Conference

NCAA D3

University of Wisconsin - Whitewater

Whitewater, Wisconsin

Great Lakes

Wisconsin Intercollegiate Athletic Conference

NCAA D3

Ursinus College

Collegeville, Pennsylvania

North East

Centennial Conference

NCAA D3

Utah State University

Logan, Utah

South West

Mountain West Conference

NCAA D1

West Chester University of Pennsylvania

West Chester, Pennsylvania

North East

Pennsylvania State Athletic Conference

NCAA D2

West Virginia University

Morgantown, West Virginia

Mid East

Big 12 Conference

NCAA D1

Western Michigan University

Kalamazoo, Michigan

Great Lakes

Mid-American Conference

NCAA D1

William & Mary

Williamsburg, Virginia

Mid East

Colonial Athletic Association

NCAA D1

Winona State University

Winona, Minnesota

Mid West

Northern Sun Intercollegiate Conference

NCAA D3

Yale University

New Haven, Connecticut

New England

Ivy League

NCAA D1

Chapter 10: What Exactly Is A Specialist In Gymnastics?

Specialist is a gymnast who is a specialist in a specific event instead of competing in across all events of the All Around. If a gymnast competes in only rings will be known as the rings specialist. It is a common practice for the male sport of gymnastics. The specialists typically (but not necessarily) have more complex abilities and perform routines with greater proficiency than gymnasts who are all-around.

Gymnastics Risks

Injuries are one negatives to participating in acrobatic gymnastics. those between 11-15 are most susceptible, based on research conducted at University of Sydney. University of Sydney and published in the issue of May 2010 in the magazine "Physical Therapy in Sport." Acrobatic gymnastics is a sport where individuals perform the sport in groups of. The results of 73 interviews with gymnasts who acrobatics were found to have 50.7

percent had suffered a gymnastics-related injuries in the previous year, and 28.8 suffered from chronic injuries in the course of the research. Most commonly, the sites of injury were ankles, knees and wrist. The risk factors were higher if gymnasts were 13 years old or over, as well as if gymnasts were training for more than eight per week for more than 11.Gymnastics is among the sports that has most injuries among girls, as per research conducted done by Ohio State University and published in the April publication of "Pediatrics." Between 1990 between 1990 and 2005, 425,900 girls and boys between the ages of 6-17 received treatment in emergency rooms due to injuries resulting from gymnastics across the United States. Injuries that could occur when doing gymnastics was 4.8 percent for every 1,000 gymnasts. Gymnasts aged between 12 and 17 experienced the highest risk of injuries of 7.4 per 1000 gymnasts.

Pressure to Diet and Eating Disorders

Dieting excessively can pose an extremely risky thing for children girls. The pressure to be small for gymnastics could cause eating disorders as well as slow growth. This can have long-lasting psychological consequences for preteens as well as teen girls. In an NCAA study of gymnastics teams there were 51% of team participants who suffered from eating issues.

Gymnastics Safety

If it's the pleasure from a flawless routine or the excitement of playing with uneven bars the sport of gymnastics can be a demanding activity that's fun and an excellent way to keep healthy.

For your safety when competing or practicing be sure to follow these suggestions.

Safe Gymnastics Gear

The type of equipment required will depend upon the specific event (uneven bars or floor routines or balance beam, etc.). Security items to consider include:

*Wrist straps, guards and grips. Gymnasts of males wear them for the still rings, parallel bars, while female gymnasts put them on uneven bars. They aid in a gymnast's grip on the apparatus, and also protect the hands from blisters. The majority of grips are made up of the leather strapped to a strap for wrists. Alternative options are wrapping hands with tape, or gauze. Gymnasts, in particular novices, need to utilize grips, tape or gauze to shield their hands from blistering or tears.

Footwear. Shoes designed for the vault generally have a reinforced sole for absorbing the force from landing. A few gymnasts sport shoes that have rubber soles to prevent slippage in the balance beam.

Spotting belts. The spotting belts are connected to cables, which connect with the ceiling. They aid gymnasts when they're learning an entirely new technique or attempting to master an exercise that is challenging.

Safe Gymnastics Practice and Competition

For safety while training or competing in competition, gymnasts must:

Take a physical prior to starting any new activity.

Make sure to warm up and stretch prior to doing any gymnastics.

Practice only on padded flooring, not on a concrete surface. Mats should be placed beneath the equipment, and secure to ensure that they are secure at all times.

Have a coach or program director that is certified and present at all practices. An experienced coach is current on the most recent safety standards.

A coach should be looking out for any challenging or new stunts.

Tell the instructor that they're not comfortable when performing a gymnastic maneuver. If they're not supportive inform a parent or administrator.

Do not attempt to perform an action in the game or in a competition hasn't been practiced enough.

Be sure to follow the rules for gyms for example:

A single person can be riding a trampoline at the same moment

If jumping into a foam pit fall on your feet, the in the back, or on the bottom and avoid diving headfirst, or falling on your knees

Only one per person using the equipment (such as rings, bars that are uneven or balance beams)

There is no training by itself

Dress in gymnastic clothing which won't catch on the equipment.

No jewelry

Please refrain from chewing gum.

If they are injured or experience the sensation of pain. Gymnasts need to be checked through an athletic trainer physician, coach or nurse prior to returning to training.

You can play different sport throughout the year to help prevent injuries caused by overuse.

Be aware of the team's plans for emergency situations. For instance, calling 911 in the event of an injury to the neck, head, or back injuries, and not lifting the injured gymnast.

Healthy Gymnastics

Gymnastics can be a great means to remain active and healthy. Just like dance or cheerleading as well as ice skating, you'll feel a lot of pressure to remain fit. The gymnasts in this situation are more at risk of developing eating problems. The effects of eating disorders could lead to severe health issues.

Parents and coaches should encourage healthy eating and are aware of symptoms of eating disorders. Being aware of an eating disorder in the early stages makes it much easier for someone to heal.

While gymnastics is a game which is popular with children as well as frequent and high-impact training there's not much details on risk factors for injuries and the efficiency of injury techniques. More controlled studies are required to determine the extent to how injury prevention countermeasures are able to reduce or prevent the likelihood of injury as well as injury re-injury. A special focus should be given to improving the facilities for training as well as the development as well as testing of apparatus, personal equipment utilized by gymnasts as well as coaching, as well as the significance of spotting for the prevention of injury.

A word of caution: gymnasts competing in competitive events can be at risk of a range of health concerns, including accidents as well as eating disorders. Make sure you are in close contact with your physician to ensure you're physically, mentally and emotionally well-balanced throughout the course of your training.

Gymnastics Fees

A discussion about gymnastics wouldn't be complete without taking on the question of cost. It is a costly sport.

How much? The amount of money gymnastics can be based on your individual scenario.

Affordability

Naturally, it is possible to take steps to make fitness more accessible, but lets begin there.

The cost for gymnastics is contingent on the kind of gym or gym you're planning to join. The big, well-known and famous for-profit gyms will be the highest priced choice for gyms. Less crowded and smaller gyms tend to be less expensive options to take gymnastics classes.

The community-based gyms, for example ones in community centers, or in the local Y can be more cost-effective for beginners to start gymnastics.

If cost is an issue make sure you look for your nearest YMCA and other community centres. They often have gymnastics or tumbling classes for local young people. The majority of Y's have scholarship programs in order to provide access to all.

Recreational Fees

Each gym bill for classes in a different way, however the majority of classes are paid monthly or by session. The gymnasts enroll for their particular level of class and monthly payment is made to pay for tuition in gymnastics.

Due to the selection of gyms which offer programs for recreation, their prices is also subject to change.

Classes for recreational classes range between $25 per month for an hour each week up to $75 an hour, based on which fitness center you decide to exercise at.

Make sure you look into the various options available to you to find gymnastics lessons.

There are a variety of classes offered in the majority of areas.

Home Equipment

There aren't any pieces of equipment for home use that need to purchase, since the majority of coaches tell that you should leave gymnastics to the gymnasium.

However, do you really believe that your child may have a desire for something or all things? Certain essential equipment at home can aid anyone in their journey to gymnastics.

The first thing to consider is that a high-quality mat is vital to stretch. I suggest a mat that has at minimum 1.5" (but prefer 2") of top-quality foam.

The next thing I'd suggest is the pull-up bar, or even stall bars. Both will assist gymnasts greatly in strength and shaping gymnastics.

Team Costs

A third factor that can impact the total cost for the sport is whether or not your gymnast is going to compete.

Gymnasts get so excited every time they get invited to join the gymnastics team, or even a the pre-team (pre-competitive group). The opportunity to compete and train is huge for many kids.

Announcing that you're part of the team could be an enormous surprise for parents who don't know how to handle the possibility!

We should prepare in advance, so that we save ourselves from the shock later.

Team Tuition

Similar to the way you pay for classes at the gym and tuition, you'll be paying for team gymnastics training. It is typically paid each month or every month for during the entire year.

The cost per month of gym training is a range of aspects. It covers the costs of your time in the gymnasium. It covers the cost of your coaches and supervisors, as well as support staff and utilities, the building and equipment for gymnastics.

However, the team tuition fee doesn't pay for all kinds of aspects. Let's look at some of the extra costs you'll have to cover for your child's participation in gymnastics.

Team Attire

Every sport has its unique rules for uniforms and equipment for gymnastics, which isn't one of them.

In terms of attire, athletes generally require the appropriate team-specific dress.

At lower levels, a team-specific leo could be a tank-style. For higher levels typically, it's an extended-sleeve leotard. The leos often have stunning designs in color as well as sparkling gems. Leos with sparkles could have anything from the fabric to glitter, sequins to gemstones and crystals. In some teams, the more glitter is more attractive!

Alongside the leotard for competition, gymnasts must also have warm-ups. It includes the team's matching trousers as well as jackets. Some gyms embroider personal names as well as the team's name on their jackets, whereas some choose to use just the team's name.

There are gymnastics teams that require shoes along with the warm-ups for the team. It could be sneakers or slides based on the gymnasium.

The majority of gyms require a group bag that is purchased to ensure that the gymnasts can compete. The bag of the team usually features the gymnast's name in it as well as the name of the team.

At the time of Covid certain gymnasts are obliged to buy matching masks for the team.

Chapter 11: Gymnastics Meet Fees

One of the biggest expenses that you'll face as the sport of gymnastics are meet costs.

The fees for gymnastics competitions - seems simple you think? It's actually not so simple. But we'll start with that.

Meeting fees cover at least your gymnast's entry fees to participate in the event. There are a myriad of types of gymnastics competitions, but bigger meets tend to be higher priced generally.

Smaller events are usually held in the gym that hosts them, however larger events are usually hosted at conference centers or arenas.

Meeting registration will be contingent on a number of variables. If the meet is approved by a league or the league that will decide the fees. The intensity of competition could be a factor in the cost of a meet.

In a typical female USA gymnastics event the registration fee would be between $85 and

$125 dependent on the event's stage and the time of the season. Naturally, there are lower-cost meets, and higher expensive ones. The cost of registration for a meet could or might not comprise the gymnast's gift.

What Else Do Meet Fees Pay For?

In addition to the cost, the way the gyms charge for meet fees and other associated expenses are subject to change.

In the event that your gym bill families, meeting fees could cover just the gymnast's admission to the event, or many other things.

Did you recall how team tuition was paid for team's time training in the gym, not including coaching? The coaches also have to be compensated for their time spent at meet and the fees for meet may or could not include this. If the coaching costs for gymnastics competitions aren't included in the meet fee then they'll be charged in a separate charge.

Along with the registration fee for gymnastics events and coach fees, your fees for the meet might also cover transportation between the venue and to the meet for coaches. Coaches may have to stay in the hotel for certain events if they are participating in several days.

Your Travel

You're, of course, in charge of the gymnast's journey between home and the event. It all depends on how far the gymnastics event is from where you live it could mean that you stay over at a hotel your gymnast competes at a later or earlier session.

Unfortunately, most of the time you don't have a precise schedule for the meet until about a week before the event, which makes difficult to arrange for overnight accommodations.

One method that our gym employed was to convince parents to book the hotel for both nights with each of them having each reservation. This way, each night could be cancelled separately without impacting reservations for the following night, or cost. For example, if your competition takes place on Saturday and Sunday you can reserve Friday on one reservation, and Saturday in a different. Most often, hotel reservations can be cancelled just a few days prior to the event without penalty, which is enough time to get the hotel which meet the timetable.

In the case of travel meets, families typically travel via planes because due to the distance. This requires planning ahead, and, of course, they are much more costly than local meet.

Regionals and Nationals

If your gymnast is able to qualify for Regionals or Nationals towards the end of the season. In this case the additional cost could be due. In some gyms that require you to make a decision at night time of States whether you'll be going to Regionals in the event that your gymnast is awarded the position. You must make that choice quickly as the gymnasiums have to reserve the spot in the event that another athlete is able to be able to attend their spot.

Private Lessons

It's impossible to discuss gymnastics or money without mentioning Private Lessons.

The private lessons can be explained in a few words. Pay the gym (or the coach) for the lessons, and they will collaborate with you individually in the time frame you specify. time. This is one-on-one instruction by a professional coach. This is not a rental of the facility for private usage.

The instructor may inquire whether you've got input into the things you'd like to improve upon during the private lessons as well as if they be looking for specific abilities to work on.

If a gymnast has difficulties with a certain ability, a trainer may suggest a private class.

Private lessons are a great resource in particular at more advanced levels, or when an athlete is struggling with mastering a particular technique. Private lessons that include more spotting exercises and drills may assist a gymnast in learning their back handspring, or backwalkover on beam.

Prepare for the Cost

The cost of competitive gymnastics can be expensive There are methods to cut costs.

Parents must conduct their own study and inquire to determine if they're satisfied with the expectations of the gym's finances. That's why you should be sure to know the amount you'll need to cover the gym, how much it will cost as well as when it'll become due.

Making preparations for financial demands will help ensure seamless transition from the sport of competitive gymnastics.

S. M. A. R. T. Goals.

Specific: focus on one specific aspect to improve.

Measurable. It is possible to quantify or suggest the progress you have made.

Assignable. Specify the person who is responsible for the assignment.

Realistic - describe what outcomes can be realistically attained, given the resources available.

Time-based - state when you expect the result(s) will be realized.

It is possible to make a huge goal of becoming a top gymnast seem easier to manage by break it down into smaller goals that are more manageable. Make goals for your training that are precise, achievable and achievable, as well as relevant and time-bound.

In this case, for example there could be the goal of achieving level 5 before the end in the calendar year. This can be broken down into smaller objectives like working on a particular move at the bars for a specific quantity of times each week, or mastering your split jump before the end of each month.

A coach is able to assist you in setting realistic and useful targets for your exercise in relation to your strengths and the level of your skills.

Self-care is the best way to stay healthy and avoid burning out. Being a gymnast at the top of your game is quite challenging and it's very easy to become exhausted and lose a enthusiasm for the game. To prevent it from happening make sure you take care your body and mind. The ways you can take care of your self include:

Spending time in the company of supportive family members and friends

Eating healthy meals

Sleeping well

Enjoying a relaxing time, like reading, watching TV or doing projects that are creative.

Talk to your doctor or a nutritionist in order to keep an appropriate diet. The right diet can be a challenge when you're training to become an elite gymnast. Discuss with your coach, medical professional, as well as a nutritionalist or dietitian regarding the food you must eat to maintain the weight you carry in a sustainable method and obtain the nutritional benefits that you require.

Gymnasts generally require an enriched diet of proteins and carbohydrates to stay energetic and build strong muscles while training. But, the type of diet you'll need may differ based on the type of training.

Be sure to take in a variety of different fruits or vegetables as well as healthy fats (like the ones found in nuts, fish and seeds as well as vegetable oils) to ensure you get all the minerals and vitamins that you require.

Request a financial aid grant to fund education.

Training in competitive gymnastics is extremely costly. In addition to the training, equipment, tuition as well as other costs along with costs for your family, you will be paying anywhere from $3,000 to $15,000 in a year. If you're not able to finance the cost of your gymnastics training, consider applying to grant programs, like Acrobatic Gymnastics Foundation's Athlete Assistance Grant.

If you're uncertain what you should do, inquire with your instructor if they could aid you.

If you're not eligible for grants, think about soliciting funds from relatives or friends via crowdfunding platforms like GoFundMe as well as MakeAChamp.

Pro Tip

Do not set so many objectives that it's difficult to determine which goals are the most important. It will feel as if you're doing nothing, and it's likely that you'll find yourself overwhelmed. Set up as many as one big goals and about 1-2 smaller objectives or three small ones.

Create an inventory of the people and the resources that you'll require for achieving your objective. This will help you become focused on the actions that are necessary to reach the goal.

Make a list of important milestones along the route to reach your goal. Each milestone can be paired with rewards. Small rewards can keep you motivated.

If setting a SMART target doesn't work for you, think about creating an open goal especially for exercising at the beginning of your journey. There's always the option of setting goals that are more specific later!

Chapter 12: The Mental Meltdown

You is getting in the morning, at 7:15am early on a cold, wintery morning. All week long, you've been energized to be more efficient at gymnastics prior to this day you've decided to get up earlier to put your equipment on take your gear bag to head right into the gym for a workout on the pommel horse technique. However, now that your day is here... You realise that it's Saturday. It's cold the body is aching after yesterday's workout as well as being comfortable and cozy on your couch at this time to rise and begin your training. Then you hit snooze to set your alarm clock and fall back to bed.

What became of the enormous amount of Motivation that you have?

Let's not be too hung up on, athletes have to deal with these issues often and under certain conditions, it's fine to rest a bit. In the end, competition brings many strains to the body and demands some recovery and time. The problem only arises in the event that skipping training and being unable to stick to your obligations becomes a routine. Unfortunately, this is and, I'm talking about very frequent. Take a look at some of the pledges that your peers and friends make during summer... "I'm going to lose 20 pounds and get my body summer ready... I'm going to diet and eat nothing but fruits and vegetables for the next two weeks... I'm going to wake up early every day and go to the gym."

Then, a couple of months later, and you know what? Nothing has changed! There is no diet, there's losing weight as well as of course, none of the early morning workouts. In order to get there with a lack of determination, it is very difficult to get the things completed. When you're an athlete, this can make all the difference. For you to succeed in gymnastics it is essential to determine the motivation behind your actions in order to take it into consideration and utilize it to drive your effort.

Definition & Examples

Motivation: Your "reason", your "why" of what you are a slave to and the things you strive to achieve.

Example

1. "I'm staying late after practice today to work on my grip and endurance." What's the reason I'm staying up later? because I'm trying to become more athletic than my brother. My motivation lies in doing better and beating my brother.

The Little-Known Facts The concept of motivation can be a great deal deeper than that, so here's a brief overview. There are two kinds of motivation... Intrinsic motivation and extrinsic.

Intrinsic Motivation: motivation which is derived from your own inner self or comes from within you.

Example

1. "I am a fanatic and a passion for gymnastics. I do not require any additional

recognition from anyone or particular prizes to continue competing and I just love being a part of the game."

Extrinsic Motivation: the motivation is derived from an outside source. your own.

1. "I enjoy competing in gymnastics since the sport makes my father content. Additionally, for each competition we win, our team am rewarded with a crisp $20 note which keeps me motivated to do my best.

The Game Plan

Simple distinction right? If you're not sure of the distinction between these two types of motivation, please be sure to read all definitions and examples. Perhaps you are contemplating which motivation can be the most effective for maximising the potential of your abilities and effort? You may have guessed Intrinsic Motivation You are right. Here's why.

If the motivation you feel comes from within, you don't require a reward from outside or any kind of reward to push yourself and put in your best effort. This is something that's from within, and there is burning within you to never stop pushing your limits. There is a burning passion and a passion for gymnastics and when you do get something in the process, it's great to be recognized, but it's not essential to keep pushing yourself. In fact, it's how very successful gymnastics athletes stay at the highest levels of performance. While watching your favorite sports stars on TV, it's not easy to see since they're in the spotlight and get all the attention of their fans but what's not seen is the countless and countless of hours of work taking place in the background. It's not surprising that the most talented athletes are also the ones who last quit the gym even though they know they're superior to everyone other athletes.

However, on the other side in the event that an athlete has a high level of Extrinsically Motivated, they could be able to achieve success at initial stages... However, what happens eventually is that the motivation begins slow to diminish, that results in the athlete "burning out." If you're not aware of the concept of Burn Out, it's simply the term used to define the mental and physical fatigue experienced by athletes. How can this be the case? This kind of athlete also has a hard work ethic and only does it to get a reward. They work to earn the prize is a hard worker for the award, and works to earn the cash. After the athlete has acquired the external items that he or she wants to achieve What happens following? What happens next? What's the reason behind their continuing to put in the effort? NOTHING! There's no reason or motives for wanting to constantly improve and become better. The sole motive of this individual was the desire to earn an external reward when it's placed within their reach, they're in a state of comfort, smug and unmotivated. In the end it's not a problem being recognized for an sporting achievement...it's in fact something that you should be satisfied with and deserves to be recognized. This is only evident when your primary objective is to be the top.

What's the lesson to be learned? To be a success at gymnastics, it is essential to identify the motivation that drives you to succeed. Find the reason. Find the reason. Be sure to choose something that is a source of happiness for you and not some other person. Make sure to keep that flame in your the longest time possible as once it's out of your system, it's extremely difficult to keep it back up and running.

Mental Workout

1. List all the reasons you choose to participate in gymnastics. What's the reason you compete? Is it Intrinsic or Extrinsic?

2. Note down the main motives for why that you are motivated on one occasion then feel unmotivated the following day. What kind of distractions are in your life? What can you do to keep them from getting impeding your achievement?

3. Discuss your experiences with colleagues and friends to look for why they are

motivated. Are you able to identify which people are intrinsically motivated as well as who is Intrinsically Motivated?

Goal-Setting

Mental Meltdown

Imagine the following scenario... You get after a lengthy nap only to find yourself in the car without a cell phone, or other technological gadgets in sight. It's a long drive to a small town you've heard lies to the north of where you are, however you have no clues on what to do in order to get there. There's no way to tell what distance this area is and how long it'll be to reach it.

What do you have to do?

It's a bit absurd (as there is a good chance that you won't get to be in that situation) However, it illustrates the point perfectly clear: can't know exactly where you're going without a clear road map! A goal is just it's a plan that will help you reach your goal of achievement. However, due to some oddity the majority of young sportsmen have no intention to set clear and precise objectives. That leads to the question... What do you want to go? How do you arrive? What time will you arrive? What information do you require in order to be on time?

The best athletes know what they are looking for, are aware of precisely what they need to do to reach their goals and also what it will take for to reach their goals. It's not an extremely difficult method to grasp, but there are some key factors that you should be aware of when it comes to of learning the right goals-setting techniques. When you have these techniques in place then you'll be light years ahead of the competition and dramatically increase your odds of success!

Definition & Examples

The goal is the final result of a goal you have set or attempting to achieve.

Example

1. "My goal is to be the best gymnastics athlete I can be."

A majority of the objectives you have set to yourself are likely identical to that of the scenario earlier. It's very simple, extremely simple direct to the point. There's an issue in creating goals this way. Why is this? This kind of goal doesn't be achieved! They don't get achieved since they don't provide a way to measure the progress made. The setting of a broad goal will not give you an ability to monitor whether you're moving forward or backwards or if you're in the same position. This is a simple fix that will require the athlete to become more precise. This brings to the following point...there are two kinds of categories with regards to goals: short-term goals as well as long-term goals.

Long-Term Goal - Your principal goal/target. (big picture)

Short-term Goals - points which must be met in order to reach your longer-term goal. (small scope)

Example

1. "Two years from now, I intend to improve my weight capacity so that I'm able to lift to my maximum of 40 pounds. This is my goal for the long term. To accomplish that goal, I must increase the weight I am able to squat to my maximum by 20 pounds per month. This is a rise by 5 pounds each week. Those are my goals for the short term. To boost my weight that I'm able to lift to my maximum of 5 pounds per week I'll be doing squats every two days after practicing and monitor the number of sets I complete in addition to the amount of weight I'll be able to put on the bar (even with more specific short-term objectives)." It's the more precise your measurements the more accurate you will be.

Week 1

Monday Tuesday Wednesday Thursday Friday

Three sets of four reps each at 140lbs. Three sets of four reps

140lbs 3 sets of repetitions

145lbs

Overall = increase of 5lbs

Week 2

Monday Tuesday Wednesday Thursday Friday

Two sets of three reps

The weight is 145 lbs. 2 sets of 4 repetitions

at 145lbs. 3 sets of two sets of 2 reps

150lbs

Overall, 5lbs more weight gain.

Week 3

Monday Tuesday Wednesday Thursday Friday

Three sets, 2 reps each at

150lbs, 3 sets of 2 sets of 2 reps

150lbs 2 sets of sets of 2 reps

155lbs

Overall, 5lbs more weight gain.

Week 4

Monday Tuesday Wednesday Thursday Friday

One set of 2 sets of 2 reps

150lbs two sets of 2 reps

150lbs 1 set of 1 rep at

160lbs

Overall, 5lbs more weight gain.

The Game Plan

Okay let's quickly recap. It is important to establish an objective for the long-term (destination) as well as short-term objectives (specific direction) that will help you achieve the level you want to achieve. Simple. Now let's go one step farther. When you decide to set either a short or long time goal, you must ensure that it's too Easy however it shouldn't be too challenging. The difficulty level that each goal must fall within lies in the moderately challenging category. Look at the following spectrum.

Chapter 13: Goal Setting Level Of Difficulties

Too Simple- It's not at any time challenging

Very Easy - Just one or two things that can be a bit challenging

neutral- An equal equilibrium between challenging and easy for you

Moderately challenging- challenging and challenges your limits

It's too difficult- Extremely demanding and hard to see the real changes

The formula that works is in the middle of the difficulty range because of the fact that such goals are challenging and will test your abilities, yet they give the conviction that you'll be able to accomplish the goals you've decided to achieve. Consider the flip facet of the coin. If a task is too simple, it does not stimulate or inspire you. This can lead to boredom. Likewise, when the goal is exceedingly challenging, it's very difficult to get any improvement or outcomes. In the absence of any outcomes or improvement, your faith will fall to the floor, which could eventually result in you stopping or giving up. This is the last thing we need to do.

Last but not least, a thing that is essential to remember for the rest of your life is that every when you make a plan will be to include the following features. The acronym stands for"SMART.. It stands for:

Specific: Every goal you decide to set should be precise, concise, and succinct.

Achievable: any objective you decide to pursue must include an element that can be measured. If you're trying to get more efficient, you can track yourself and if you're looking to improve your strength you can monitor the amount of weight you're able to lift.

Aim-based: any goal must be a call to steps, physically or mentally.

Realistic- As we said in the beginning, your objectives must be achievable (in the moderately challenging category but not impossible to accomplish or even incredibly simple).

Every goal has to be backed by a time limit, an appropriate timeframe that will ensure that you're doing what that you can in order to meet the goal.

There you go you have it, you have the Proper Goal Setting Methods. Through integrating all aspects of Long-Term Goals as well as Short-Term Goals as well as the Goal Setting Difficulty Spectrum and SMART...you will be able to boost your performance up to a top level in a fast rate. Keep in mind that as you get closer to achieving the objectives you've established, the process will get simpler and more straightforward for you, and allow you to alter your goals over time that will help you become more effective as an athlete.

Mental Workout

1. Start now and write down three long-term goals you'd like to achieve.

2. Plan out an outline of short-term targets of the way you'll achieve those three long-term targets. Keep track of your progress on a regular basis, whether weekly, daily and even a every month.

Mental Imagery

Mental Meltdown

There's nothing better than going to see one of the thrilling and classic gymnastics films. They range from Peaceful Warrior, to Nadia The Truth Behind The First 10, to Gymnast, American Anthem, Stick and the list could go on for a long time... The point is that there's something when you watch a film on the sport that you are passionate about that inspires you to go back into the training facility and keep working hard! This could be because most of us subconsciously or not, we put ourselves into the roles of the primary protagonists in the film. We ride the emotional rollercoaster that the movie depicts... We feel the sadness, we experience the pain, are frustrated but at the end we experience the joy and triumph when the movie characters unite and achieve victory against Adversity.

In reality, this procedure is what mental Imagery (also called Visualization) operates! Mental Imagery is similar to watching a film within your mind just pressing the play button on your DVD player when you're ready.

In contrast to the films reality is that things aren't always the way you'd like them to. If, for instance, you've had an embarrassing game or being up to par, it's possible to reflect back and consider through all the mistakes that you've made in the course of the game or throughout the whole season. Imagine yourself making a few errors, ignoring your plan and not adhering to your game plan, becoming angry, being yelled at or being mocked as well as losing your spot in the team, despite all the effort and hard work. You end up in a major "funk" which is the exactly the opposite of what you were hoping for in the beginning! To stop such a scenario It is essential to recognize that the thoughts that you create in your mind are extremely powerful and have a profound influence on the performance of your gymnastics. Knowing how you can use mental Imagery is crucial as it is essential to utilize it for your benefit rather than a hazard to gain the advantages.

Definition & Examples

Mind Imagery (Visualization)Utilizing your imagination and thought processes to produce extremely detailed images and photos within your head. The images could be of memories from the past or of future ones according to the way you'd prefer them to unfold.

Example

1. I'm at the back of my yard, performing my backward squat. I close my eyes, and visualize myself doing the routine, and then preparing my turn. I lean down and there is an uproar I can feel the tension, yet I'm comfortable. I

push my body upwards by bending my legs. I then spring up, kick my knees upwards and push my arm back, forcing my body to spin around, then I fall exactly in the floor. The crowd is roaring, my friends have a blast jumping up and down in excitement. I feel the excitement coursing through my veins. It's a flawless flip!

The Game Plan

If you're hoping to become the best gymnastics performer in the near future, you've likely turned your back and thought of achieving massive results during contests... concerning executing your routine flawlessly performing your routine to get the perfect scoring... of achieving amazing comeback victories .... as well as gaining the respect of your family and colleagues. It's normal and the best athletes all do regardless of the sports they compete in. It is important to understand that the method by which you think about these mental images has to be executed effectively and efficiently way. You may be surprised to learn that there's a specific method to doing this. This is a checklist of the components you must utilize to bring mental imagery for your athletic career to maximise your abilities.

Prior to you begin your workout routine, before you lift weights, prior to participating in an event live and anything else that demands the use of a particular skill or procedure, you should take 10 minutes to visualize succeeding. Imagine yourself doing it correctly with every move, every motion and each step. Imagine each time you jump off the vault, you perform your leap perfectly and smoothly, being confident and technically strong that other athletes start to think they won't beat your strength, and being so solid that any weight you set on the bar is to be light. It's like you're bursting with confidence and you're able to take on anything that is thrown at you. While you're doing this it is crucial to remain extremely, and by that you mean extremely detailed and exact about the scenes the images are running through your mind. As I said earlier that it's as if you were playing a movie your mind.

It is essential to use all of your senses: touch hearing, smell and smell, taste. Once you've learned how to integrate all of your senses into one, you'll be able to see how you become more like you are in the exact moment you're thinking about. That's our goal. As you imagine vivid, detailed mental images your brain releases exactly the same chemical and messages throughout your body just as if there in that exact instant. It will enable for you to feel exactly the same reactions and phenomena you'd experience when it was happening in real-time, permitting you to plan beforehand and offer the sensation of "You've been there before" as the time comes to experience that moment.

Example:

Imagine that in your competition yesterday, you did not perform quite well on the uneven bars and particularly the gienger release, and finished last. It is likely that you could do far better. So, before next week's event, take 10 minutes to imagine yourself doing your best with your gienger releases. .... "I go between my hands, grasping the bar at a high angle using both hands. I feel the cold sweat splashing onto my t-shirt I can feel the cheers of the crowd calling for an upcoming fall. I feel and smell popcorn from the bar that serves snacks and my gaze is fixed to the bar. I build the energy... as then I perform my normal procedure... move up, let go of the bar using the left side of my hand. I reverse flip then slowly spin... It is then that I turn through mid-air before locating the bar using my eye's corner and extend my arms. grab the bar again by both hands, then seamlessly transition into the next move...picture flawless execution." Then repeat the procedure over and over again each gienger...elevating your self-confidence each step of your process.

The process of becoming more proficient in using mental imagery may be demanding at times due to the fact that it's not something that can provide quick positive results. Therefore, it's essential to understand that, just as with all other skills you've acquired, it will only gain proficiency with dedication and consistent practice. As a child and you started learning walking, it didn't happen in just one day. It required weeks or months, to master the ability to perform every step properly. Don't be discouraged or angry during the initial stages of mentally imagining even when you don't feel it's doing the job. Practice, and keep improving, and over time, your ability can be greatly improved.

Mental Workout

1. Learn the techniques in the final paragraphs. Choose a subject you would like to master prior to practicing, or during your practice visualize yourself becoming successful. Imagine yourself performing everything correctly. Make sure to focus on the details and think about all actions, the

steps and all the things that is happening around you.

2. When you've mastered the art of your mental imagery works for you, begin developing routines. There might be a place with a calm atmosphere to go or a tune you could download to your Ipod or an exact time of day that visualizing can be more efficient for your needs (in the morning, when you awake, or in the evening before you sleep). Do this as often as is possible. Write your routine down.

Chapter 14: Thought Suppression Mental Meltdown

The balance beam is in view and all eyes are upon you as the time slowly ticking as the clock ticks. The time is nearing the conclusion of your workout and all you need to do is end your workout with a strong performance for your team to be in the best chance of securing an impressive win, and secure the chance to compete at the national championships. But...as you take your final steps and begin an handstand...you're your body's weight is slightly tilted to the left. This breaks the focus of your body for only a single seconds. Then you try to compensate by shifting your dismount in the very last moment, but you ultimately, you fall off of the beam...completely damaging the routine you've just put together. The round is lost and the team forfeits the championship. When you get home on the bus, you're unable to help but think of that same thought running over your mind...

"I DON'T WANT TO THINK ABOUT IT ANYMORE!"

It can happen to even the strongest of us...all we would like to do is put this unforgiving experience in the most dark and mysterious nook of our brain and lock the memory away for ever...never to return. It is our goal to stay as far as we can from these overwhelming, traumatic feeling of anger, despair and despair.

The process of thinking is known as thought Suppression and precisely the kind of thing that athletes indulge when they have a bad performance. However, does Thought Suppression an effective strategy? Does Thought Suppression the most effective method of overcoming a performance that isn't good? What happens when you are turning off your thoughts? In reality, Thought Suppression is mentally one of the most harmful things to perform when seeking to boost the performance of your athletes. This is akin to doing nothing before a huge exam, and you're creating a risk for yourself to fail.

Definition & Examples

Thinking Suppression - trying to stop yourself from thinking about an idea or trying to prevent particular thoughts from being a part of your thoughts.

Example

1. We can further look at the scenario that was discussed in the preceding section. Your balance has slipped and you've dropped on the final loop and now you're in a long trip home on a bus. It's the similar thoughts "DON'T think about it Don't think about it! !"

The following day is here and you're still doing to avoid thinking about the incident. For your own benefit You try something slightly differently... each time your thoughts about falling to the ground resurface in your thoughts and you try to replace them with different memories that are disconnected and without any connection. It's like thinking about the delicious tastes of your favourite food...you imagine your fun coming family vacation...and you contemplate the way that those brand new Jordan sneakers fit you. (things which usually make your body feel healthier)

Guess what What? Here's where things become somewhat confusing because the first thing that happens is that your uncomfortable memory of falling gets a connection to the good memories of food or your trip with the family and even your new Jordan sneakers. This means that each when you consider these wonderful memories...your thoughts return to your balance slipping and falling!

It's not easy to grasp how this happens at first, but it's an extremely common phenomenon that is referred to as the Rebound Effect.

The Rebound Effect of Thought Suppression when you try to block the thought (not even think about the thought) however, you will get into the habit of being thinking about it more. The mind is occupied contemplating the exact idea you're not going to be thinking about!

The Game Plan

As it's a concept that is contradictory we'll explain it in more in greater detail. Memory functions within your brain is through creating links between related things or thoughts. In the example above, if somebody mentions the word "dog" what automatically pops in your mind? Then you'll probably begin to think about "paws, bark, bite, and fur." The more strong the connections are between these items or concepts and the more likely you have of recalling those particular memories. Since your brain doesn't discern between unpleasant memories and enjoyable memories and pleasant memories, by blocking your thoughts and trying to replace a painful memory with a more pleasant one, it's actually creating a link between them. It's important to know as a gym person or any athlete for that matter since "DON'T THINK ABOUT IT" frequently leads to the complete opposite of what you want to achieve. purpose is...which would be to recover from the embarrassing or poor performance incident. It begs the issue.. If the decision to not think about it does not bring about the desired outcome What can you take to help over your mistakes?

There are numerous options available, however one stand out over other options ....and it's known as the Mindfulness method. It is possible that you have heard the concept of Mindfulness during your beginning career, perhaps even seen it on Television because professional athletes are gradually recognizing the benefits of Mindfulness. Sam Mikulak (seven time NCAA Gymnastics Champion) is an incredibly well-known figure who utilizes mindfulness practices to enhance his performance when in contests. Many books and articles have been written on mindfulness, and numerous research studies have shown the benefits that it has, which are recognized by sport associations from around the globe. To get to the point however...Mindfulness is simply a word to describe a state of mind where you allow yourself to experience any and all thoughts you have and simply choose to view them in a non-judgmental manner. The ability to acknowledge that your thoughts are not negative or good, they are an inevitable part that is part of our lives. It allows you to live every moment fully as well as take whatever happened. Particularly in the field of gymnastics, it is important to accept that there will be a variety of ups and downs. any athlete will be subject to this, no matter the level of their performance. There will be mistakes and it is not recommended that be allowed to derail you while you attempt to progress in your professional career. If you're prone to Thinking Suppression, be conscious of it and adopt the Mindfulness approach to your thinking method. The experience you have as a gymnastics player will improve and become far more productive.

Mental Workout

1. The next time you participate participating in a contest, make an effort to track the thoughts that affect the performance of your competitors. Note these ideas in the space below.

2. Look at your list above. Do you think these thoughts are a result of bad experience that you've faced previously? Explain.

3. How can you apply the Mindfulness method immediately to prevent you from suffocating your thoughts?

Competitive Anxiety

Mental Meltdown

The day you've been waiting for only a few minutes away. Everything you've put into throughout the season is now in the balance. Every single hour of training, your early morning exercises and late-night filming sessions and the sweat, the blood and tears, suffering, agony and defeat...all that has led to the moment you are in. The championship for the division.

What are you experiencing? Sweaty palms? Are knots or butterflies forming within your stomach? Do you find it hard to loosen up and stretch? Do you find yourself looking upwards at the stadium you realize how many will be watching you play? Do you feel the pressure of this event?

Whether you're in a youth league or in the pros... young or old...a rookie or a veteran...competitive anxiety is experienced by every and all athletes at some point in their careers. While experiencing a few anxiety before a match is normal, there will be times when athletes are so stressed that anxiety takes over their thinking process, which results in a significant underperformance.

What exactly is this thinking method? For starters it is the result of internal phobia. Fear takes over the mind of the athlete, and these thoughts generate fearful feelings, and the fearful emotions result in fears that trigger actions. This is a vicious cycle that's difficult to break. With the proper attitude and practice, you'll be able to reduce the chance of feeling high levels of stress and anxiety during the times that matter most for you and your team.

Definition & Examples

Competitive Anxiety- that anxious sensation you feel prior to the big event, or during an important moment in an event, or even after the event. The most common cause of anxiety in competitive situations is an idea in your head which you're "expecting" to happen, and this specific thing makes you anxious to the point of being.

In addition to Competitive Anxiety There are two common results, fear of Failure and choking under Pressure.

1. Fear of Failure: an enormous fear of risking with your life, fear of failing and a fear of moving beyond your comfortable zone, fear

of failure or being successful, and of the consequences that could result.

Example

a. At times, at the conclusion of a practice session, coaches might require one player to complete the drill within a specified period of duration. If the workout can be completed on time then practice ends for all. If the exercise is not finished on time, everyone has to follow up with other conditioning drills. Are you the one who takes the initiative to do your part and do you slip back and do not wish to face the demands? Are you worried about what might happen when you fail to finish the exercise within the timeframe?

2. Choking (Choking under pressure)Not being as efficient than you typically are. Gymnastics is a sport where choking crucial times is typically related to blowing an enormous lead, making minor mistakes in your routine, sliding during the last few seconds as well as "shrinking" or shying away at the most critical moment of competition.

The Game Plan

What can you do to keep anxiousness about competing that could ruin your gymnastics program? What can you do so that you avoid the dread of failing that is preventing you from achieving your goals? What can you do to avoid being a victim in moments when the most important thing is to you and your team?

First thing to be able to identify what is that you are afraid of What causes you to be scared as well as what it is that causes you to perform poorly. The most frequent factors that contribute to higher levels of anxiety about competing may seem surprising to you: your friends or family members, as well as your coaches and teammates. What causes this? Most young athletes get obsessed with what the view of other people would be if they did have an unsatisfactory performance. What, for instance, would your peers discuss at school in the morning in the event that you fall off the pummel horse at the end of the round? How upset will your family members be in the event that you choked on the exercise on the floor and didn't have the chance to put your team in the lead? What would it be like going to the practice the following day, knowing your team and coaches were furious when you failed to follow the game's plan of attack and failed to perform as planned? If you've had these thoughts running through your thoughts at times, don't to fret, you're certainly not all alone! The most important thing to remember is that these scenarios is actually true! Yes, I'm going to say this again, they're not actually happening. These are just thoughts that cross your head, all arising from...yup that's right... Fear. If you stopped worrying about the implications and instead concentrated on the job that you were tasked with, the reaction within your body would totally shift. The outlook will in turn reduce the anxiety that you feel.

Sometimes there are athletes who experience an anxiety or fear of failure or even scream when under stress because of one of these experiences previously. This is a differently because the moment a similar incident occurs the same thoughts come back, bringing together all of the negative emotions and thoughts that had previously pushed athletes into doing poorly. There's another difference to be recognized to change the results for the athletes. And here it is...Instead of thinking of past failures as obstacles, as insurmountable mountains, as impossible challenges...athletes should instead think of those failures as opportunities to learn, as chances to correct a mistake, as a second wind to blow past the competition. This would alter their thought method, and that's what makes all the distinction. All it is is a matter of the perspective. Only you can lose if accept that you will fall. Every loss you make will be an opportunity you can take away, and applying the lessons learned to your next steps is essential to achieve the success level you want so much.

Mental Workout

1. Make a list of your top three Olympic gymnasts. Go online to see what kind of obstacles and adversity they've faced through their entire career. Have they received criticism? What are the issues they have struggled with? What have they done to help?

2. Ask yourself the same questions that you asked above. Have you ever been the subject of criticism? Have you had any issues? How did you respond? Based on what you've learned today, how do you react differently?

Chapter 15: Self- Talk

Mental Meltdown

"How did I become so dumb? Why didn't I do it even when I had a chance? What is the reason I keep continuing to train despite the fact that it seems as if I'm never getting better? It might be time to stop?"

The above questions represent the moment when an athlete has hit an obstacle and is forced to criticize themselves to the point where it is totally ineffective. If it's because of an unsatisfactory performance, committing an error in competition or even making an oversight when they practice...athletes throughout all sports have such moments because they're almost inevitable, yet challenging to conquer. There is hardly anything accomplished by trainers and coaches to rectify these self-deflections that can make it very difficult for an athlete to acknowledge that they have a problem and an unforgivable practice that doesn't work in their best interests. This unwelcome problem and behavior is a direct adverse effect on an athlete's ability to perform at their best.

The issue is easily solved by mastering the skill of mental thinking (yes it's a thing) that is Self-Talk. In contrast to what many might believe...Self-Talk is proven to be a strong psychological ability that's employed by some of the top athletes in the world. There are some important distinctions that must be considered, and we'll begin by delving into what exactly Self-Talk is, and then break it down into two distinct kinds.

Definition & Examples

Self-Talking: talking to yourself in public or within your head.

It's very simple. But, in order to make sure that athletes aren't evaluating themselves or their performances These two kinds of self-talk are now commonplace.

Positive Self-Talk: Telling yourself phrases, words, and affirmations that will motivate you to stay on track with your goal.

Example

1. When I am getting ready to perform my show on the ring I remind myself that "No one can beat me." "I'm too strong." "I can easily win."

2. "Hard Work Beats Talent When Talent Doesn't Work Hard" is a common quote.

Self-talk to instruct yourself: telling yourself the rules to ensure you're meeting your expectations.

Example

1. If you're getting at a point where you are able to do the 1/4 turn of dismounting from the beam, you could say to you "transition to a handstand remain strong and lift my left hand off the beam. Do a counterclockwise rotation and place it on the floor." This is exactly how the coach will instruct the procedure during the practice.

The Game Plan

It might seem odd to you that an insignificant change to how you perceive and react to your personal behavior and outcome can have significant changes to your performance in sports. In reality, however, your words have a lot of power and can have an impact on your perception of your world. Particularly when you start thinking about what to do when faced with challenges and how to get through important moments in your life as well as how you can keep pushing when the fuel tank is full of fumes...self-talk is a great resource. An excellent example of this is none other then Annie Hilton, a highly gifted young gymnast from Temecula, California. If you're not aware of her tale, at just ten years old, she was struck by a severe neck injury as she was preparing her routine to make it onto the US National gymnastics women's team. For added complication doctors found out that Annie had dyslastic spondylolisthesis. It's a condition that prevents her vertebrae joining. The experience was horrendous and necessitated the need for a complicated, painful surgery. You can imagine it was an extremely lengthy recovery process which was a real test for her mentally and physically.

You can guess...one of the most important psychological skills she rely on to aid her rehabilitation process was self-talk! If you're able to research her story, make sure you do as it's an inspiring read. It's been reported that she said during certain times, she'd tell her self "people need to take care of all things for me. I'm not able to take a walk by myself "... "It's very difficult to feel weak. "... "What distinguishes me from other people is that I'm unique is the fact that I'm adamant "... "I am going to get back to be stronger than I was prior to." Slowly, her thoughts took an improvement... She changed her mind to believe she might have been injured to the point of death and then believing that she had the potential to resume the sport at a high standard. In addition, she was successful in her return, but she also defied chances by regaining her fitness and winning national championships and again.

Finally, regardless of whether you prefer the concept of the positive or instructive self-talk method I would suggest to combine both and neither one is superior to each other. If you can develop each of these abilities, you'll gain a significant advantage over the competition. They will improve your capacity to remain concentrated, which is an essentially missing art in our modern sports arena. Additionally, it's advised to begin developing an "script." A script which you can refer to whenever you're feeling like you require more confidence, or a boost to overcome any difficulty you are facing. The script you create can be derived from any source, and you could create it by yourself or search "Motivational Quotes" and you'll come across a variety of simple sentences that will help you stay focused and inspired. There's one thing for sure, you're bound to deal by many challenges during your time as a gymnastics player there's no doubt about that. It's essential that, the times that challenges arise when they do, that you're prepared for these challenges with the right tools to allow you to conquer and overcome.

Mental Workout

1. Write down 10 phrases, words and affirmations to keep focus. It is possible to use any thing you've seen on a screen or in a magazine or read in a novel It could be something that a person has said to them, advice from your teacher, any other thing you'd like. You can mix it up.

2. Set yourself in a competitive circumstance and look at ways to utilize self-instruction. Note down the instances of what you might think to yourself. Note as many instances as you possibly can.

Zones of Optimal Performance

Mental Meltdown

Think about a time when you watched your favourite gymnast excel at a elite performance. The list goes on and on. Simone Biles winning four Gold medals at the Rio Olympics in 2016 to Kerri Strug battling through injuries to take home the Gold Medal in 1996, to Paul Hamm making an incredible winning comeback in 2004, (just to mention a handful of) There have been numerous shows where gymnasts leave spectators in admiration and awe. It seems like every difficult move they perform is flawlessly performed, each step they take is able to provide the needed movement and standing that allows them to seamlessly transition during their performance it appears like they're one step ahead of the rest. What do these amazing feats share to do with each other, regardless of who's taking part in them? If you attend any of the interview sessions after the performance, you'll definitely be hearing them talk about...

"I was in a ZONE."

Attaining the "Zone" is one of the top goals for every athlete, regardless of what sports they take part in. It's an attitude that allows everything flowing in their direction and everything seems to be effortlessly and easily. Gymnastics athletes talk about the comfort of playing the sport. Winning competitions is like stealing candy from a child as every movement becomes silky smooth. It's an amazing thing to watch...and isn't it more thrilling if you, as an athlete could learn how to reach this state of mind? What to be able to recreate this experience repeatedly? Sure, your performance in contests would increase dramatically! Our goal is to help you take from these tips to aid you in determining the place where your performance zone is to ensure that you achieve the required skills to achieve this state of mind.

Definition & Examples

Zone of Maximum PerformanceThe level of stress which you are at your best reaching an "mental zone", reaching an optimum state of mind, in which everything seems to flow effortlessly and you are to the highest level physically.

Chapter 16: Attention

Mental Meltdown

The time has come for competition! The sound of the bell goes off and you're the winner of being the first to rise in the initial round. However, within just a few seconds the whole thing goes to hell! An accidental slip in your exercise on the floor can result in an easy deduction of points, and after recovery, your whole routine is off-track. Once you are back on the right track, you are preparing for a body-slide that is sure to return any points you've forfeited, but as your feet are positioned again on the floor you begin to lose your balance. It's your attempt to stop yourself in time to avoid falling, but you're too late, as is the case with another points deduction by the judges.

In the time of a gymnastics contest, it's a massive array of activities happening all in your vicinity simultaneously. It's possible to practice as many as you can however, nothing beats competing in a live event. It is essential to keep in mind each and every aspect of the routine the coach instructed you on during your practice. You must to be quick in recovering from emotional breakdowns, and you must be able to be prepared if you find yourself losing control or your balance. You need be aware of how your score can impact the scoreboard as well as standings. You need to be aware of the adjustments you'll have to make to be successful the game, and all the way to. It's a challenge to keep track of everything. It's not even mentioning that everything is happening as your coach yells at you from the sandbox while your friends and family have been screaming towards you in the crowd as well as your teammates seeking your attention, whether they're present on stage or sitting on the bench. When there are so many competing for your attention, you're like a sniper in zone of war and you must concentrate all your attention to the issues that matter to you at the time.

Definition & Examples

Diverse Attention- trying to focus on several things at a simultaneously (multitasking). Since your attention is split it isn't performing better than when you paid full concentration to one area at the same moment.

Example

1. Balance beams are among of the toughest tasks for every gymnast. It's challenging because the decisions have to be taken in just only a few seconds, your attention must remain focused only at the beam and your game plan has to be thoroughly known as your plan will change depending the position you're on the ladder (first spot vs. last). The focus must be laser similar, because a single error can result in an unintentional slip and tumble, leading to an unsatisfactory result.

is a. Inattentional Blindness- This word describes the phenomenon of the inability to recognize something quite easily apparent (obvious). The thing you aren't able to notice is due to your inattention. concentration.

Example

1. Your coach may instruct you to execute a particular jump in the vault round then you are enthralled about doing that exact jump. It's still rings round, but your inattention to the event leads you to fall short. Everyone will see that your head is elsewhere. However, you're so focused on getting your task that you fail to think about or see anything else that's happening within your vicinity.

The ability to discern irrelevant information while focusing on most important information.

Example

1. As you sprint towards the table to vault, you should be focused on your jump and removing any distractions, while concentrating on performing your leap correctly.

The Game Plan

This diagram provides an excellent illustration of how the mind could serve as a filter, or funnel when you compete. Think about it this way: you execute an array of difficult actions, and the audience is enthralled by it, and you are convinced that the judges will give you an impressive score, however you wind with a low point score. The worst part is that you're further back in the rankings and must gain space to move up. When this happens, it's easy to become distracted and have your mind split in the direction of how you could've gotten more points or how you could have done things differently. What you need to be paying attention to is scoring a higher score in the next round! It's that easy. But so often, athletes are caught up in being concerned about how poor the judges are or what kind of trash others are speaking about or how fans are rude. When athletes are distracted by all the stupidity and different situations instead of being present in the present, they're underperforming and are subsequently dismissed. Beware of this.

www.ingramcontent.com/pod-product-compliance
Lightning Source LLC
Chambersburg PA
CBHW071442080526
44587CB00014B/1951